NEW DIRECTIONS FOR MENTAL HEALTH SERVICES

H. Richard Lamb, *University of Southern California*
EDITOR-IN-CHIEF

A Pragmatic Approach to Psychiatric Rehabilitation: Lessons from Chicago's Thresholds Program

Jerry Dincin
Thresholds

EDITOR

Number 68, Winter 1995

JOSSEY-BASS PUBLISHERS
San Francisco

A Pragmatic Approach to Psychiatric Rehabilitation: Lessons from
Chicago's Thresholds Program
Jerry Dincin (ed.)
New Directions for Mental Health Services, no. 68
H. Richard Lamb, Editor-in-Chief

Microfilm copies of issues and articles are available in 16mm and 35mm,
as well as microfiche in 105mm, through University Microfilms Inc., 300
North Zeeb Road, Ann Arbor, Michigan 48106-1346.

LC 87-646993   ISSN 0193-9416   ISBN 0-7879-9946-6

NEW DIRECTIONS FOR MENTAL HEALTH SERVICES is part of The Jossey-Bass
Psychology Series and is published quarterly by Jossey-Bass Inc., Publishers, 350 Sansome Street, San Francisco, California 94104-1342.

EDITORIAL CORRESPONDENCE should be sent to the Editor-in-Chief,
H. Richard Lamb, Department of Psychiatry and the Behavioral Sciences,
U.S.C. School of Medicine, 1934 Hospital Place, Los Angeles, California
90033-1071.

Cover photograph by Wernher Krutein/PHOTOVAULT © 1990.

TCF Manufactured in the United States of America on Lyons Falls
Pathfinder Tradebook. This paper is acid-free and 100 percent
totally chlorine-free.

CONTENTS

EDITOR'S NOTES

There are three components in psychiatric rehabilitation. Each is necessary, and each can act independently of the others. However, for psychiatric rehabilitation to work best, all three should act synergistically, each strengthening the other until their sum is greater than their single efforts. These components are medication (Chapter Two), the rehabilitation relationship (Chapter Three), and rehabilitation program efforts (Chapters Four and Five). This volume, *A Pragmatic Approach to Psychiatric Rehabilitation: Lessons from Chicago's Thresholds Program,* deals with all three, assessing their importance and explaining how they can be integrated in comprehensive psychiatric rehabilitation. (Although more pages of this particular volume are devoted to program efforts than to the factors of medication and rehabilitation, I ask the reader to bear in mind that all three factors are equally important and interactive in program members' rehabilitation.)

The example used throughout this volume is the program approach at Thresholds, a Chicago-based agency for psychiatric rehabilitation, and all the contributors to this volume hold or have held important staff roles at Thresholds as managers or program directors. The Thresholds approach is essentially pragmatic and practical; it is based on what works. Thus, the description of Thresholds' specific program direction and orientation is supplemented by discussion of its special program efforts for specific subsets of program members. In addition, Chapter Six describes the outcomes of Thresholds programs as evaluated by the Thresholds Research Institute over many years, Chapter Seven examines administrative issues that I see as important in agency growth, and Chapter Eight introduces a number of issues that all practitioners in this field ought to be discussing more frequently.

While this volume focuses on the Thresholds example, my colleagues and I do not feel that the Thresholds approach is the only or the best approach, or even the recommended approach. There are many ways to help the mentally ill, many program styles and philosophies. Yet, since our field lacks a large number of robust comparisons of approaches, we tend to bolster and support our personal evaluations of what is the best program. This is natural and as it should be. Rigorous experimental designs are seldom implemented, often unproductive, and typically constraining to the immense creativity rampant in our field. So, "Let a thousand flowers bloom," as Mao Tse-tung once said, and let all participants, including staff, members, and leaders, taste the fruits of their good sense and labor. Anyone who claims to have the "correct" or patented approach or who argues that psychiatric rehabilitation should hew to a single philosophical or programmatic line does this field a disservice. Many approaches are valid and will work. This particular volume describes one that has evolved over thirty years and that makes sense to me.

NEW DIRECTIONS FOR MENTAL HEALTH SERVICES, no. 68, Winter 1995 © Jossey-Bass Publishers

There is no "right way" to do psychiatric rehabilitation. The Thresholds way results from what we think we can do for and with our members, while being appreciative of the expectations of our funding sources, responsive to local and national conditions, and alert to expansion opportunities. Though ours is not the only psychiatric rehabilitation model, it has been effective for us, operating well on a practical level and supported solidly by practical results and research. Of course, like any pragmatic approach, ours is subject to change. This volume, then, contains the contributors' current thoughts on psychiatric rehabilitation, illustrated by the story of how and why Thresholds operates and how it arrived where it is today.

I wish to acknowledge the help of Judith Cook, who partially edited and commented on this volume and, especially, the assistance of Kathy Robinson, who typed and retyped my many drafts with unfailing good humor. In addition, I want to thank all the many former and current Thresholds staff who have not authored a chapter but whose presence is felt on every page. Our various government funders, board of directors, contributors, and of course, our long-suffering members also have my sincere appreciation.

Jerry Dincin
Editor

JERRY DINCIN is executive director of Thresholds.

Agency history, basic principles, and attitudes influence
a comprehensive version of psychiatric rehabilitation.

Roots, Fundamental Ideas, and Principles

Jerry Dincin, Dale Bowman

Pencil lines etched on a closet wall in Thresholds' first building once marked the year-to-year growth of the children in the former home of Pulitzer prize–winning author Margaret Ayer Barnes. Early Thresholds staff left the markings from 1892 and 1893, idiosyncratic reminders of the past. We all leave markings on the places we visit and the people we meet. Thresholds, Chicago's first psychiatric rehabilitation program, has left its share in the thirty-five years since its opening on February 11, 1959, at 1153 North Dearborn in Chicago's Near North neighborhood. While that graceful brownstone no longer hosts a stream of former mental patients playing games and participating in groups and while the pencil markings in the closet surely disappeared years ago, the memories remain. The markings left by Thresholds and its staff are outlined in this volume.

Beginnings

The foundation of the Thresholds approach to psychiatric rehabilitation is the clubhouse program that characterized Fountain House in New York.

In the late 1940s, a number of discharged mental patients began meeting on the steps of the New York Public Library for fellowship, calling their group We Are Not Alone (Dincin, 1975). An association of concerned women then provided Fountain House, so named for the fountain in its courtyard, to give these former mental patients a better place to meet. After a tight ruling clique used a heavy and controlling hand to include and exclude members, the group nearly dissolved into anarchy. However, the 1955 appointment of John Beard as executive director changed all that and brought a sense of professionalism into the agency. Beard made the vocational component central to programming, and it remains central at Fountain House today. Moreover, instead of becoming a clinic where former patients could come for infrequent medication adjustment and occasional counseling, Fountain House adopted a clubhouse approach that developed a sense of belonging in former patients. Being a "member" of a club rather than being a "patient" in a clinic is more than a change of words. "Membership" connotes people's involvement in the life of the club and responsibilities for its operation; it designates a safe place for members to develop friendships.

The influence of John Beard and Fountain House on the development of the program at Thresholds has been profound. From the day I walked into New York's Fountain House in June 1958, my thinking on psychiatric rehabilitation grew and matured and my life changed dramatically. As a professional social worker in his first job, I was paid $4,800 per year, but the salary was far less important than the opportunity to get involved in what clearly was a good cause. It also helped that Beard was a maverick; that appealed to the persuasive, competitive, and rebellious sides of me. I loved working there. I took from him the pleasure of innovation: the inner delight and self-righteousness of demonstrating that there is a better way than conventional wisdom. I truly care about getting good things for people with a psychiatric illness, and these were stimulating times in which I learned a great deal about the basics of psychiatric rehabilitation.

In 1963, I became executive director at two of Fountain House's tiny branches in New Jersey (later named Friendship House and Prospect House). In September 1965, I became executive director of Thresholds. During my next thirty years in that position, I used my Fountain House training and also moved in many different directions that made sense to me.

When I arrived in 1965, the program operated with four full-time staff and me, plus a student intern, a business manager, and a secretary, and a budget of less than $100,000 a year, with monies coming from the Illinois Department of Mental Health (DMH), the Chicago Community Trust, and the National Council of Jewish Women (NCJW). Thresholds has always had a diverse array of funding sources, and this situation continues. No community fund raising was done then, and it was hard to recruit board members. To convince people to serve on the board, we actually had to promise not to ask them for contributions. In 1970, our expansion into the rooming house next door at 1155 North Dearborn enabled us to convert the upper two floors into housing for members and thus began our first small residential program. In 1972, we purchased a building at 2700 N. Lakeview for our main headquarters; then we had to overcome strong community opposition to move there. One neighbor filed a lawsuit that effectively delayed our moving into the building for several years. Fighting the fears of the community and the stigma of mental illness has been one of Thresholds' constant battles.

Over the years, I helped and nurtured Thresholds' growth from that handful of five professionals operating primarily a social center for released mental patients to over 450 staff running a psychiatric rehabilitation organization that serves about 3,000 people yearly in seven district day program branches plus thirty sites for various styles of group living arrangements, operates with a budget of $25 million, and offers comprehensive services for its members, people with a history of hospitalization for mental illness.

Thresholds had its genesis in 1957 as a project of the Chicago chapter of the NCJW, whose members wished to "sponsor a program of activities and counseling designed to develop the social skills of former mental patients as part of their rehabilitation in the community." As part of the planning process, an NCJW member (Pauline Penn, who remains a Thresholds board member) visited Fountain House to see how it functioned.

Threshold's first official day of programming, in February 1959, was attended by three clients and two volunteers (Curina, 1959a). By March, Thresholds was serving seven members three sessions a week. The March report of the first executive director, Maryann Curina, showed that members were dealing with many of the same issues they confront today (Curina, 1959b). From members' fairly consistent social, housing, vocational, academic, and health needs, as well as the overarching need to prevent unnecessary hospitalizations, the six goals (described in Chapter Four) of Thresholds gradually emerged. Meeting these goals became the basis for Thresholds programming.

The 1950s saw the beginning of serious use of medication for the treatment of mental illness. Huge numbers of patients were being deinstitutionalized owing to the use of psychotropics (introduced in the United States in 1954). In 1958, 57,000 beds were utilized in state mental hospitals in Illinois. In 1994, the number was about 3,200. While deinstitutionalization was initiated by the use of medication, it was spurred by humanitarian aims and concerns about patients' civil liberties. But there were additional economic and political reasons: it was less costly to house patients outside of hospitals in nursing homes and intermediate care facilities (ICFs), and the owners of these homes and ICFs were a powerful political force. Not much thought went into what would happen to patients after they were deinstitutionalized.

The idea of released patients coming into a social setting on a daily basis was "radical thinking in those days," according to Ed Goldman, Thresholds executive director from 1963 to 1965 (E. Goldman, conversation with the author, Oct. 1993). Thresholds, with its informal nonclinical atmosphere, encountered much resistance from the professional psychiatric community. The early opposition centered on the fact the agency was not headed by a psychiatrist. An early board member, Sylvia Astro, then on the faculty of the School of Social Service Administration at the University of Chicago, remembers that "it was an era heavy on the psychoanalytic approach and anything less was looked upon with some doubt" (S. Astro, conversation with the author, Sept. 1993). Some professionals outside of Thresholds would have liked the agency to close up its party and become another clinic. In fact, Goldman sometimes ran into trouble obtaining funding because he insisted, with the backing of the board, on maintaining Thresholds' direction. He was also to be instrumental in introducing the prevocational component into Thresholds programming. After visiting Fountain House and John Beard; Horizon House and Irv Rutman in Philadelphia; the Center Club and Sam Grob in Boston; and Hill House and

Hank Tanaka in Cleveland, Goldman obtained some funding for an employment program from the Illinois Division of Vocational Rehabilitation. The DMH funding gradually increased (Bond, Witheridge, Setze, and Dincin, 1985).

"We set the basis in Illinois for what would be called psychiatric rehabilitation," Goldman recalled. "It was based on social skills and vocational rehabilitation, rather than a clinic. In those days, that was a radical, radical departure and thought to be on the fringe. I or the agency could not have survived without support around the country at other similar places."

One of the appeals of Thresholds was that people could walk into 1153 North Dearborn and always find something going on. Small groups were meeting, discussions were occurring, people were playing pool or Ping Pong. No one else in Chicago was doing the Thresholds' style of programming in the early 1960s, but similar agencies were sprouting and surviving around the country. Goldman's description of his years at Thresholds could serve as a general description of the early years of psychiatric rehabilitation around the United States: "In overview, members in general were better because of what we were doing. We were the only agency open on Sundays. Even in the early days, we weren't a 9 to 5 program. We were successful not on the basis of dramatic individual stories, but because of a lot of little success stories."

Some of the basic philosophies of Thresholds existed early on. The strong emphasis on the social aspect of rehabilitation existed from the first day. The vocational side began developing in the early 1960s. Both remain central to Thresholds' psychiatric rehabilitation. The bottom line at Thresholds has always been transitioning members out of the hospital life into a decent life in the community. However, when I came to Thresholds in 1965, I felt that this transition required a more comprehensive approach. I was not pleased with the existing program emphasis and behavioral expectations. There was not enough rehabilitation going on, and what was available had a Freudian psychoanalytic overlay that was not sufficiently rehabilitative and was unacceptable to me. To make a long angry story short, the board of directors was forced to choose between my rehabilitative Fountain House approach and the more analytic emphasis of the rest of the staff. In November 1966, the board chose my approach, the remaining staff resigned, and from that point forward, the agency's programming was rebuilt to emphasize fifteen underlying principles. These principles help us frame our ideas and daily work. Our basic tenets of psychiatric rehabilitation evolved over the years, changing in response to different locations and the needs of different populations, but all used our unique style of rehabilitation as summed up in the following principles.

Fifteen Underlying Principles of Psychiatric Rehabilitation

Comprehensiveness. Services in a psychiatric rehabilitation center should be as comprehensive as possible. This is Thresholds' most basic principle of doing psychiatric rehabilitation. Services should not be parcelled out to other agencies. It is not effective to have vocational services provided at one agency, residential services at another, a day program at a third, and medication prescription at a fourth. That splitting up of member needs is ultimately very confusing to the member, encourages one agency to play off and blame the other, and most importantly, creates a climate in which bad communication is inherent, with the result that members easily fall through the cracks created.

Another advantage of comprehensiveness is that it adds flexibility: members of an agency can add to or change their rehabilitation program as warranted. A member's program may focus at the beginning on medication and staying out of the hospital, then shift to stabilized housing or social concerns, then move on to vocational and general health concerns. If one agency is doing the job, staff and members can focus resources where they need to be at the time they are needed. Those engaged in psychiatric rehabilitation must remember that agency members are trying to piece together lives that have disintegrated. Offering whole and complete services makes the job of reintegration easier.

Sense of hope. Sometimes agency members do not have an active sense of hope. Without that sense, they slide into despair, a very difficult hole from which to climb. Both the agency environment and staff, in particular, need to engender a sense of hope. If staff feel hopeless, members will not feel necessary energy or hope. The sense of hope is an essential part of rehabilitation. Without the idea and belief that change is possible, nothing will be changed or improved.

Sense of pride. A sense of pride derives from a sense of accomplishment. Whatever staff do in psychiatric rehabilitation should be done with the serious intention of instilling a sense of pride within the member. Because staff are often forced to carry the sense of pride early in the rehabilitation relationship, they must express genuine pride in what the members are accomplishing. Often, this expression means reframing members' achievements so members can understand and appreciate them. In the end, the pride staff feel will lie in members' taking pride in their own lives and recovery, in their rebirth of new life.

Sense of belonging. One of the crucial advantages of psychiatric rehabilitation over other forms of treatment is the sense of belonging. Because members are in a clubhouse setting, they become part of the clubhouse. It is theirs, and they develop a sense of belonging similar to that found in other sorts of communal living situations, such as sororities and fraternities. It is not the same as belonging in a familial setting, but it is a sense of community that imparts a strong sense of acceptance. It also builds a sense of participation.

Without members who belong, psychiatric rehabilitation could not exist; it would be a party with no guests. Members have the crucial part in their psychiatric rehabilitation, and they must seize an active role in it. Participation in their own rehabilitation is their most important task.

After the trauma of being psychiatric patients, members need to recover and get their lives in order. The reason they go to a place like Thresholds is to make improvements, whether small or large, in their lives.

Sense of responsible control. The sense of responsible control often lost by patients in mental hospitals can also be absent in members, particularly when they are in the throes of a symptomatic regression. When members exercise a sense of responsible control, it is usually a sign that they are getting better, especially when they can sense internally that they have this control.

In the psychiatric rehabilitation arena, no one is talking about a cure or even sees one on the horizon. What we are all looking for are ways for members to function within the confines of the symptoms of their illness and to make the best of their lives.

There probably will always be some loss of potential in the future of members' lives, which needs to be addressed with love, understanding, and directness in the rehabilitation relationship. What psychiatric rehabilitation tries to achieve is recovery to the greatest extent possible, recovery to each member's highest functioning level. This recovery must be accomplished at least partially through the reduction of symptoms. That means taking prescribed medication properly. The sense of responsible control begins with proper medication management and gradually grows into a stable life-style.

Behavioral orientation. Thresholds places strong emphasis on helping members change their behavior. It is patently clear that a member must learn to function in the community and to establish normal social relationships. Insight, per se, is not the primary goal; it is a secondary tool. The notion that positive behavioral change must be preceded by insight is rejected by psychiatric rehabilitation.

Experiential approach. At Thresholds, in keeping with the behavioral principle just described, we believe members learn through experiences, and therefore we provide a wide variety of learning opportunities, which may be chosen by the members based on their own desires or staff suggestions. Experiences that help members learn how to relate to one another and to their co-workers on a job assignment are prime examples of the experiences offered in this approach. The way staff assist members to prepare for job interviews, by conducting several mock interviews and coaching members on how to respond, also reflects the experiential and learning nature of psychiatric rehabilitation.

Pragmatism. One characteristic that marks all psychiatric rehabilitation agencies is a pragmatic emphasis on helping members with the practical problems of living. Rehabilitation does not involve any academic approaches. It works on reality, on what needs to be addressed now and on such longer-term practical issues as a job, housing, and improved social life.

Regression. Although regression may be an inevitable part of the lives of many of members, from the point of view of rehabilitation, it is not a positive experience. The strange notion that psychiatric patients will emerge stronger and better if psychotic episodes are simply allowed to run their course is not accepted. There is simply too much pain and disorganization in the psychotic process. Thresholds does not encourage regression or feel complacent about it. Staff work to stave off regressive tendencies and to keep people functioning.

Successful experiences. Many members have told Thresholds staff that all they needed was "a little self-confidence." That is probably the single most common statement made by members to explain their need for a psychiatric rehabilitation program. Helping to create a self-confident person is an arduous task and one for which no therapeutic modality has an exclusive license. Thresholds staff feel that the creation of a number of small successful experiences is one of the ways to build a more confident person. Since all of the members have failed in one or more of the important functions in life, they need a rebuilding exercise that slowly, in steps as small as layers of snowflakes, increases their level of confidence. Our ability to make successful experiences happen for members is the most creative way that all of us use our programming.

Appropriate milieu. A milieu must exist in which staff and members can effectively tailor the activities offered by the agency to fit the unique needs of a member. The availability of a great many program components and the ability of staff and members to emphasize one aspect over another are important strengths of the rehabilitation approach. Combining programs to suit the levels of many different people is a creative exercise in the use of milieu, and one that has been honed to a high degree of therapeutic efficiency at Thresholds.

Almost any visitor to Thresholds will remark about the sense of hopefulness, the feeling of activity, and the expectation of improvement that seems to pervade the atmosphere. Exactly how these impressions are transmitted to members and visitors is hard to describe. The important program characteristic of a strong expectation that the members will be involved, for example, echoes the belief of many in the field that activity can absorb anxiety. However, the quality of that activity also is important if this expectation is to be communicated. Thresholds strives to make activities meaningful, and toward this end, staff constantly evaluate and reshuffle activities and programs. Meaningful involvement is doing something purposeful that is not emotionally deadening.

Member choice. It is a basic tenet that the member has choices. Members' active involvement in their own rehabilitation essentially becomes the respect that members have for themselves. It is the member's life, after all, and he or she has to live it. So members' choices are crucial and, in the final analysis, must be respected.

Parents and relatives. Parents and relatives often form the strongest support group for members. But they also have suffered secondhand damage from the family member's illness. Parents and relatives are so important that Thresholds established a Parents/Relatives Group (discussed in Chapter Eight).

Parents are sources of vital member information and of solid histories of members. After the onslaught of mental illness, the family is often a member's only surviving social network. Parents and relatives must be utilized and included in the rehabilitation process as much as possible.

Hierarchy and informality. Reducing the basic hierarchial pyramid is imperative in psychiatric rehabilitation. While there are branch directors, program directors, and team leaders at Thresholds, we *all* try to maintain active contact with members and with the milieu at each location. In any setting, there is some degree of hierarchical control. Ultimately, someone must make decisions, but the distinctions and levels of hierarchy in a psychiatric rehabilitation agency can be deliberately blurred to create an informal environment. The hierarchical structure can be far less clear cut than in a medically oriented facility for instance. The setting should never have an institutional look or feel to it. This is particularly a given with in vivo approaches, such as the assertive outreach model used by Thresholds Bridge programs (described in Chapter Four). The feel of an informal setting includes staff and members calling each other by their first names, staff actively participating in agency functions, and staff and members forming softball and basketball teams together and, most importantly, playing together.

Dependency. There is much that is positive to be said for dependency. It is unwholesome dependency that is worrisome. Often, Thresholds staff attempt to transfer an unwholesome parent-child dependency to the more wholesome dependency that develops in a staff-member relationship. This we feel is positive growth. Dependency per se is not necessarily bad—being something everyone has to some degree and being, indeed, a stage that members may need to go through. But at the same time, staff encourage much independent member action in community adjustment.

These fifteen underlying principles in psychiatric rehabilitation must be organized within in a particular framework of components if their application is not to be a case of "the devil is in the details."

At Thresholds, there are three of these framing components. The first is a belief in the biological basis of mental illness and its impact on the rehabilitative program. The second is a respect for and belief in the power of a rehabilitation relationship between member and staff. The third is the actual program at Thresholds, including all the efforts in social and vocational rehabilitation, the housing operation, and the academic studies and physical health areas. When the actual program and actions that result from a belief in biological causes and in relationships are combined with the philosophy described above in the fifteen principles, Thresholds emerges.

References

Bond, G. R., Witheridge, T. F., Setze, P. J., and Dincin, J. "Preventing Rehospitalization of Clients in a Psychosocial Rehabilitation Program." *Hospital and Community Psychiatry,* 1985, *36* (9), 993–995.

Curina, M. Unpublished memo to heads of area mental health organizations. Thresholds, Feb. 1959a.

Curina, M. Unpublished report to the board of directors. Thresholds, Mar. 1959b.

Dincin, J. "Psychiatric Rehabilitation." *Schizophrenia Bulletin,* 1975, no. 13, pp. 131–147.

Jerry Dincin *is executive director of Thresholds.*

Dale Bowman *is manager at Bargains Unlimited, a branch of Thresholds.*

Belief in the biological roots of mental illness will govern
some of what we do in a psychiatric rehabilitation program.

The Biological Basis of Mental Illness

Jerry Dincin

No tenet of psychiatric rehabilitation holds more importance than the centrality of the biological basis of mental illness. From this basic understanding
stems the focus on preventing hospitalization via medication compliance. The
understanding of the role of biology in mental illness is important not only in
and of itself but also in combating the stigma attached to mental illness and
the resulting frequent denial of mental illness by rehabilitative agency members. At Thresholds, the response to the centrality of biological causes is three-
pronged: medication education, medication prescription, and medication
compliance.

Biological Illness Requires Biological Treatment

The definition of mental illness that I gave in a 1989 speech in Miami and later
adapted for a *Psychosocial Rehabilitation Journal* article still holds validity for
me: "most mental illness starts with a genetic defect, accidental or inherited,
which predisposes a person to a significant bio-chemical disturbance in brain
neurotransmitter functioning. An extremely low tolerance for stress, either of
biological or psychological origin, can trigger the exacerbation of symptoms,
but is not itself causal. This altered biochemistry leads to distortions in 'normal' perceptions, emotions, behavior, intellect, and other brain functions that
collectively we term 'mental illness.'"

Without this change in brain biochemistry, we would not see the symptoms we call mental illness. Therefore, it is absolutely basic that we try to
restore a more "correct" brain chemistry so that symptoms will be reduced and
members' behavior will return to what our Western culture has decided is
"normal." This restoration is accomplished through the intelligent, sensitive,

knowledgeable administration of medications that help correct brain chemistry gone awry.

Occasionally, perhaps too frequently, medications are prescribed by people without sensitivity to the member or to the side effects the medications cause. Sometimes, they are administered by mean-spirited and punitive personnel. Sometimes, they are administered by people without intelligence or caring. I make no defense of these people except to say that sometimes symptoms are so disruptive and outrageous (which of course is not the "fault" of the patient) that heavy medication and/or restraints seem the only course possible. Poor administration is never excusable and must be corrected by careful monitoring of personnel and their attitudes, habits, and behavior. However, even the overuse or misuse of medications does not change the basic truth as I see it: mental illness is essentially biological and almost always needs to be corrected by biological means (in other words, medications).

At this point, the best thinking of scientists I respect indicates that mental illness lies in some defect in the dopamine and/or serotonin systems. And it appears dopamine receptors are the key to understanding these defects. Although there are five receptors, the two most important are D-2 and D-4 and their interactions with the serotonin systems. Although all this is subject to change as science brings us more insight, what we do know now is that medication works: it affects those dysfunctional sites in the brain. What we do not know for sure and what we need to keep an open mind on is this: is there a developmental error or a gap in early neurological development and, if so, is the cause a genetic malfunction, as suggested in my definition, or a virus or something else.

What is also not yet well understood is the interaction between biology and psychology. That is, what is the effect of psychological trauma on brain biology? Perhaps for some people, the psychological trauma inherent in sexual and/or physical abuse or other environmental harm is so severe that it actually changes neurotransmitter chemistry in the brain. Although the jury is still out on that issue, we need to take this possibility seriously and be willing to alter our treatment protocol accordingly. Perhaps a lesser reliance on medication (although I expect that some would be beneficial) and a greater reliance on psychotherapy, hypnosis, Holotropic Breathwork, and psychosynthesis are in order for persons whose symptoms emanate from sexual abuse or other psychological trauma. Another question is whether street drugs like PCP and LSD can cause mental illness. I believe that although they can mimic schizophrenia, the effects of these drugs are transient unless the drug user is biologically prone to schizophrenia.

Of course, a person can have genetic defects and therefore mental illness to a slight, moderate, or severe degree, just as is the case with other illnesses. But at psychiatric rehabilitation centers, staff rarely see people with mild cases of schizophrenia. They see people who are at least moderately and usually severely and persistently affected.

Why is it so important that we have a causation hypothesis of mental illness? It is our understanding of the cause of mental illness that tells us what to do about that illness. Our rehabilitation program flows out of our hypothesis. If we believe schizophrenia is totally psychological in origin, caused by familial interactions in childhood, then the remedial course of action will be some form of psychotherapy. However, mental illness has been with humanity for a very long time. And from earliest recorded Western history, people with mental illness have suffered for their bizarre behavior. They have been excluded from towns, depicted as passengers on a "ship of fools," whirled in revolving chairs, chained, bound in wet sheets, and burned as witches. In more modern times, insulin shock, psychoanalysis, Laingian therapy, vitamin therapy, and lobotomy have all been tried, with modest or no effects. Electroconvulsive therapy (ECT) definitely does help some people but can have devastating side effects and is now used less frequently. The only treatment in the history of mankind that has shown consistent scientifically verifiable improvement over placebo is the use of the medications currently available. Nothing even approaches the consistent usefulness of medication in reducing the symptoms of this devastating illness. We do not know how to cure it, but we do know how to make the symptoms tolerable for most people.

As discussed in Chapter One, medication has been the single most potent force in emptying the hospitals from their highest use in the 1950s to the present. If not for the discovery of antipsychotic medications, is there any serious doubt that these hospitals would still be crammed with patients? Nothing else made a significant difference. Civil rights cases and exposés of inhumane hospital treatment, the family movement, and mental health legislation would have had little if any effect on the mental hospital population if medication had not made it possible for the heretofore intractable mentally ill to leave these institutions successfully.

Therefore, I believe that mental illness exists and has existed for all of recorded time. I reject the views of Thomas Szasz and his supporters, who deny the existence of mental illness. Nor do I believe that psychiatrists and the medical profession invented mental illness. History tells us that it has always been with us in both mild and severe forms. While it is true that some cultures revere those whom we would call mentally ill, in Western culture the symptoms of mental illness are regarded as aberrant and undesirable.

The acceptance of the biological understanding of mental illness leads us directly to the first goal of psychiatric rehabilitation: keeping people out of the hospital. For psychiatric rehabilitation practitioners, acting on this goal boils down to helping members understand the need to take medication and then actually taking it. No amount of talk therapy, group therapy, or visits with a psychiatrist will repair a biological problem in the brain. The biological side *must* be attended to as the first step in rehabilitation. Everything in a comprehensive psychiatric rehabilitation program like that at Thresholds flows from that premise. My experience has taught me again and again that many, if not most, hospitalizations are preventable. Yearly studies at Thresholds verify this observation. Forty to sixty percent of all rehospitalizations of Thresholds members are in some way related to a failure in medication compliance. Reduction of the compliance problem will dramatically reduce hospitalizations.

Issues in Medication Compliance

Members have many reasons for not taking prescribed medication: denial of illness, medication side effects, poor self-image, medication ineffectiveness, a feeling of "I'm well now," and particularly among members in a manic phase, enjoyment of the symptoms of the illness.

Each of these reasons (and the others listed later in this chapter) needs to be addressed with members. Most importantly, staff must assist members to understand that medication compliance is central to their rehabilitation and to building a new life outside the hospital. For us to ignore medication compliance or to let others take care of medication issues is to abrogate our responsibilities as caring professionals. Sometimes, I think agencies that do not pay close attention to medication issues, either for philosophical or practical reasons, believe there is no such thing as mental illness.

By the time the members at Thresholds begin psychiatric rehabilitation, they are no longer in the early stage of mental illness but usually have had many episodes and frequent hospitalizations. Staff owe it to these long-time sufferers to help them adhere to their prescribed medication. Obviously, the majority of members have the final say in whether they take medication. But staff need to be persuasive in teaching members about medication, and to be persuasive, staff must know what they are talking about from a moral and a scientific perspective.

While it is not impossible to work with people who are not taking medication, if they are very symptomatic they tend to gain little from the program. In a very few situations, Thresholds will terminate a member if his or her symptoms are so severe that it is obvious staff are wasting their time and the member's time: for example, a member whose full-blown paranoid or manic symptoms are intolerable or whose behavior is so destructive that he or she cannot function in the Thresholds community. At such times, staff may initiate or encourage hospitalization, change to another type of programming, or tell the member he or she cannot stay in the program as it is structured. But these situations are the exceptions to the rule. Exclusion from Thresholds for medication noncompliance happens rarely.

There are at least three major problems with psychotropic medications that are not yet resolved.

First, any medication that affects brain chemistry to control the symptoms of mental illness will also have secondary effects. Even mild secondary effects are uncomfortable, and the more severe ones can be unbearable. Part of psychiatric rehabilitation is to help the member decide whether the basic effect of the medication on the symptoms is worth the discomfort of the secondary effects. Most of the time, it makes sense to lean toward supporting the basic effect of the medication, since too often the alternative is hospitalization. However, this basic decision is not ours, but the members'.

Because side, or secondary, effects are a plague for members and are the single most important reason for members discontinuing their medication, they need to be taken seriously by mental health professionals who are knowledgeable, alert to their occurrence, and able to act as advocates with the prescribing psychiatrist in those cases where members cannot express themselves adequately or are unaware of the side effect. A regular screening for the side effect of tardive dyskinesia (TD) should be performed by psychiatric rehabilitation line staff, who should then report any slight TD symptom to the psychiatrist for further evaluation. Side effects are *the* major problem in medication compliance.

Also, pharmaceutical companies need to continue their efforts to invent medications that will target the precise symptoms of mental illness with fewer secondary effects. Indeed, this has happened over the years: clozapine, Risperidone, valproic acid, and Prozac are all significant improvements over prior medications. Personally, I am continually grateful that pharmaceutical companies have come up with all these improvements since 1954, and I hope they continue to do so.

Second, every person's reaction to medication is idiosyncratic as to the most effective medication or combination of medications and the correct dosage. And every person's reaction to secondary effects is different. This makes the administration of medication subject to trial and error, a kind of scientific art form. Medication should be administered by experts who keep up with the scientific literature and yet are willing to make intelligent, humane "guesses" at what is best. Amateur practitioners (family doctors) are usually not well suited for this task, but psychologists could and should be trained for this important responsibility. Finding the right combination of medications to control symptoms and control side effects over an extended period is a difficult job.

Third, known medications unfortunately do not work for some people, or they work only modestly or engender an allergic response, leaving people with too many symptoms to operate effectively. This is as sad as the situation of people with severe infections who cannot tolerate any antibiotics. Just as frustrating is the situation of the people for whom medications work well initially but then lose effectiveness over time (in the film *Awakenings,* Robert DeNiro touchingly portrayed the tragedy of temporarily effective medication). Again, we must turn to the pharmaceutical firms to keep working on this.

Program for Medication Compliance

A psychiatric rehabilitation program should include a program for medication compliance. The components of the Thresholds medication compliance program illustrate the many elements that go into such an effort:

Teach the biological basis of mental illness. Members can and should come to understand the biological basis of mental illness. Group and individual education sessions geared to a simple explanation of the biological basis of mental illness help to relieve members' sense of guilt at being ill. Issues of grief and loss of potential may then arise, but they are easier to deal with than denial of mental illness, which creates a plethora of problems.

Develop a medication education class. Members should understand precisely what medications they are taking, why they are taking them, and how the medications work. They should also understand why the medications have side effects, and staff can help members process their tolerance of those side effects. The Thresholds medication group, for example, is an eight-week, one-hour-per-week class led by a social worker. Thresholds does not have a psychiatrist running this group primarily because of the expense, but a psychiatrist usually leads one class. Each session is run as a class: notes are taken and tests are given at the end of the session. All members participate in this group.

Develop an individualized prodromal pattern for every member. Staff need information on each member's unique collection of prodromes, warning signs that are yet not full-blown symptoms. Prodromes might include increased irritability, sleeplessness, or changes in appetite or personal cleanliness. Sometimes prodromes are more spectacular, such as sudden moves to other states, but usually staff want to be alert to slight precursors to an increasingly symptomatic picture. Once a person is paranoid or manic, we are no longer talking about prodromal patterns. At Thresholds, staff try to get an initial prodromal pattern during the intake process. This information is asked first of the members themselves when they are in a stable state, but by far the best source of prodromal information is parents. Other tips on prodromes can be gathered from staff, friends, and hospital records.

Work on improving the relationship between the member and the doctor, as necessary. Occasionally, members do not like their psychiatrist or do not know how to talk to him or her. These members can to be taught how to communicate more effectively with their doctor. This process sometimes requires staff participation in the doctor-member interview to make sure the doctor really hears the member's report and, in turn, the member hears and understands the doctor's report.

Use testimonials and other peer supports from medication compliant members and former members. Despite caseworkers' best attempts, members may not believe what they say about medication. However, these members may more readily listen to and respond to other members. Thus, peer support should be used as much as possible.

Use community meetings to support medication compliance. At Thresholds, community meetings of members support medication compliance, as do occasional focus groups on medication.

Analyze precisely any resistance to medication, especially denial of mental illness. In both individual and group encounters, staff need to work with members to reduce medication resistance. Basically, nobody likes to take medication for any reason. For people with a history of mental illness, the resistance is even more pointed, and staff need to help patients see the analogies to purely physical illness. Denial of mental illness is the most difficult issue psychiatric rehabilitation staff will face. While I do not have a lot of advice on this, I can suggest that one technique that sometimes leads to a breakthrough is to ask members themselves to explain the origin of their symptoms and of their multiple hospitalizations and unusual behavior, ask them to name a cause.

Offer parents of members medication education and solicit their support. Because family and friends can exert much influence on members, support groups for them should help them understand the centrality of medication compliance and the biological basis of mental illness. Parents' support can be crucial; their lack of support devastating.

Develop and use relationship. Relationship is *the* crucial factor in medication compliance. A trusting relationship between member and staff remains the best long-term method of maintaining medication compliance.

Deal seriously with side effects. Members have some important reasons for not maintaining medication compliance. In surveys of Thresholds members, as mentioned earlier, the single most important reason for noncompliance is side effects. They must be dealt with as they arise and should not be ignored under any circumstance. Members can understand taking special medication just for their side effects. In certain cases, staff will have to assist members in tolerating side effects. A useful analogy is that the treatment for certain cancers may feel awful, but it is worth it to maintain life. Thresholds staff are taught to do tardive dyskinesia screening (using the Dyskinesia Identification System: Condensed User Scale [DISCUS]) and prompt referrals to doctors are made if warranted. Staff must always be vigilant in watching for side effects.

Analyze history of noncompliance through hospital records. It is important for staff to discuss with members the prior noncompliant experiences that have led to rehospitalization. This examination may also show what could have been done differently to increase compliance.

Start a special group for all members hospitalized three or more times. This group will focus on attitudinal issues, which might include these frequently expressed member attitudes about medication:

"I feel better without meds."
"Its 'just' symptom control and doesn't effect a basic 'cure.'"
"I no longer need meds."
"Meds do not help."
"The voices said to stop meds."
"The symptoms are better so I stopped."
"I want to test myself to see if I really need the meds."
"I want to try and do it on my own."
"I am afraid of taking it for the rest of my life."
"I want to be natural."
"I can't think as clearly with meds."

In addition, patients may make statements that indicate

Fears of dependency, addiction, or loss of control
Fears of harm to body or offspring
A sense of stigma or embarrassment at having to take meds
A dislike of the idea of taking meds
A lack of understanding of the medication's preventive function
Experiences of loss of creativity
Experiences of forgetting to take all the doses
A desire to "get back" at the therapist by misusing medication
Experiences of medication interfering with sexual desire/potency.

These and other statements and attitudes form the agenda for discussion in the medication attitude group.

Give recognition to members who stay out of the hospital for a specific length of time. Every year, Thresholds throws a major party for members to celebrate those who remained out of the hospital for a year or more. On these Member Recognition Days, the members to be honored receive certificates, are publicly praised, and receive the applause of their peers. Catered food is offered, and family members, friends, and doctors are invited.

Pay attention to any substance abuse that relates to medication compliance. If substance abuse is inhibiting a member from taking medication, seek a consultation with the member's psychiatrist. Sometimes, mixing street drugs and medication matters a great deal; at other times, it does not.

Make videos of members when they are well. These videos can then be shown to members when they get symptomatic, and vice versa.

Achieve a high level of staff training and commitment to the entire compliance program. As a part of this training, discuss problems with medication compliance and techniques for achieving it at regular staff meetings.

Accompany members to their appointments with the psychiatrist. Also, employ doctors who will make home visits when necessary.

Make a written agreement with each member, at intake or thereafter, that he or she will take prescribed medication.

Make sure there are funds for medication. Have staff get prescriptions filled if necessary.

Develop the best schedule of taking medication for each member. To help members maintain their schedules, use pill boxes or other reminder mechanisms, including prepackaged medications; use injectable medication as frequently as practical (if necessary; use a visiting nurse to give members injectable medication at home); use lab tests to analyze blood levels of medication.

Role of the Psychiatrist in Medication Compliance

When working with the chronically mentally ill, our senior psychiatrist considers it essential to be connected with an agency. The chronically mentally ill person has a complex package of problems, and the person working in a private practice will find it too difficult to take these problems on alone.

Thresholds uses members' psychiatrists in a targeted manner. None are on staff salary and none have any operational say in daily Thresholds activity; instead, they are treated as consultants. It is valuable to have as much of this consulting as possible done at the agency, otherwise communication suffers. It is much easier to speak with a psychiatrist about a member for a minute at Thresholds than to wend through a maze of answering services and beepers. Of course, many members maintain their own psychiatrists, as is their option, and Thresholds staff do not attempt to change these doctors.

In a psychiatric rehabilitation program with a mandate to avoid hospitalizations, psychiatrists need to be readily available to handle emergencies. If a staff person or a member realizes that the member is beginning to reach the point of hospitalization, our doctors are never far away. Psychiatrists are also valuable for the expert training they can be paid to provide to line staff. Such training sessions can cover general medication orientation, new medications, biological causes of mental illness, medications' side effects, and tardive dyskinesia screens.

And of course, psychiatrists are valuable in helping staff maintain medication compliance and for imparting specific professional knowledge to line and supervisory staff.

Absolutely nothing is more important in psychiatric rehabilitation than medication compliance. All our pearls of wisdom, caring, and love will not be useful unless supported by an intelligent, sophisticated, sensitive, and humane medication management and medication compliance program.

Renaming Mental Illness

Finally, once the basis of mental illness is understood to be biological, it becomes apparent that a new name for mental illness would be appropriate, one that reflects its cause. I suggest *neurotransmitter/stress syndrome*. That name would be particularly helpful as a substitute for *schizophrenia*, a term that has long outlived its usefulness. *Schizo* is now used as a derogatory term for almost any behavior we do not like or want to make fun of. Insensitive advertising, television show dialogue, and street jargon have stolen the true meaning of schizophrenic and made it into a curse word. The situation is reminiscent of the former use of moron, imbecile, and idiot to describe the three levels of mental retardation, terms that then came into daily conversation as pejorative descriptions of almost anyone. Isn't *Down's syndrome* much better as a name than any of its predecessors?

The name *neurotransmitter/stress syndrome* puts the emphasis on brain chemistry and also acknowledges that stress may precipitate the effect of defective chemistry.

JERRY DINCIN *is executive director of Thresholds.*

*A special member-staff relationship is necessary for
psychiatric rehabilitation to be effective.*

The Rehabilitation Relationship

*Richard Horowitz, Diane Farrell, Jay Forman,
Jerry Dincin*

A vital ingredient in psychiatric rehabilitation is the rehabilitation relationship, and yet little has been written about it. Most of what we read in our journals has at its core an objectivity, a quantifiable aspect. That is seen as scholarly, as positive, as how we should be and how we need to be. But how do we quantify or objectify the relationship in psychiatric rehabilitation? It is impossible to define, research, and dissect this relationship fully, and that is as it should be, for there is a "magic" here. Yet this relationship is also the glue of rehabilitation. Therefore, we need to examine it as closely as we are able, to tease apart its texture and differentiate it from other therapeutic relationships.

This chapter looks at the questions, What do we need to learn about the psychiatric rehabilitation relationship in order to do it? What are the qualities staff need to establish it? What is the best combination of the attributes and styles that make it up? Supervision and mentoring are vital methods of learning about the rehabilitation relationship. Actually doing it and then talking about how one did it is vital.

At its apogee, the relationship combines staff and member willingness to deal actively with the practical side of rehabilitation with the ability to express the finest skills of a therapist. These traits are weighted to one side or the other in a changing dynamic that depends on the moment-to-moment needs of the member, the capacity of the member, and the skill of the staff member. The special relationship is a complex arrangement, demanding staff sensitivity to the member's current state of illness and creativity in using program and community resources.

When we address the needs of a member whose course of illness is severe and persistent, or whose capacity for insight is minimal, or who comes to us

NEW DIRECTIONS FOR MENTAL HEALTH SERVICES, no. 68, Winter 1995 © Jossey-Bass Publishers

after repeated and long hospitalizations, or whose ability to stay focused is limited, or whose symptoms are always present, or who "just doesn't get it," we are talking with the most difficult of our group. With these members, we focus on practical issues. Helping each member through the day, the week, and the month with as much satisfaction as he or she is capable of and, most importantly, helping him or her stay out of the hospital are crucial goals. This work especially requires attention to the unique pragmatic characteristics of the rehabilitation relationship, combined at times (but not necessarily always) with the psychotherapeutic component.

Essential Staff Qualities

Senior Thresholds staff have suggested that all staff need to possess and express certain attributes in order to establish rehabilitation relationships. They need the ability and willingness to

Help a member overcome reluctance to participate.

Take an activist stance in helping members to motivate themselves.

See members as "people," not just "clients," accepting who they are right at that moment. Inviting them to change under these circumstances is to diminish their despair and sense of isolation.

Be confrontive when necessary, offering sensitive and sometimes strong encouragement of alternatives to self-destructive or immobilizing behavior.

Develop members' feeling of dynamic hopefulness, letting them "borrow" the strength, ego, energy, and hopefulness of staff when their own qualities are dissipated.

Be invested in all aspects of members' lives, focusing on positives not deficits.

Use creativity and energy in developing options within the agency program and within the larger community.

Be tenacious in the face of symptoms, regression, hostility, and resistance, exhibiting the friendliness, optimism, and enthusiasm that consistently reaches out to members. Staff do not give up but try again. They are in for the long haul.

Demonstrate an inner sense of love, caring, and gentleness that permeates the relationship. Members absolutely know when staff care; it is no accident that some staff are especially and consistently well loved by members.

Take on variable and various role relationships in members' lives as helper, peer, task creator, boss, mother or father or sibling, or friend, depending on what is needed at the time.

Share personal history with members, as sensitively appropriate, in order to make a point.

Make frequent contact, since a staff person cannot make an impression if he or she sees a member only once every two weeks.

Maintain a sense of humor and perspective; even grim situations can sometimes be defused by humor.

Diminish hierarchy and status differentials.

Help each member feel that he or she is understood and appreciated as an individual person, not as a manifestation of an illness, sincerely tolerating unusual behavior without being judgmental.

Show tolerance not only for symptoms but for ambiguity, confusion, and foul-ups.

Know that despite everything, each member carries his or her own affirmation within himself or herself and that the "borrowing" of a staff person's affirmation is just that, a temporary loan.

Be involved in a wide range of member needs.

Have a case of "underdogitis," an inner need to help people who are less well off than themselves and who are frequently pushed around by an impersonal system.

Both like and love members. It may not be possible to like a member all the time or to love him or her all the time, but to the degree that staff can do both, their own lives and members' lives are enriched.

Be energetic, proactive, and willing to mix it up with members.

Be empathic. Members suffer and staff need to feel their pain.

Be idealistic; staff idealism primes the pump.

Be hard workers, committed to go the extra mile for a member.

Know the goal, keeping an eye on the important issues without appearing grandiose.

Listen, really hearing what is said and unsaid.

Attend to detail where both member welfare and administrative paperwork are concerned.

Roll with the punches, not getting overwhelmed by snafus, by members, by other staff, or by administrative expectations.

This may sound like a prescription for sainthood, but do not be discouraged. There are no perfect staff people, but every staff person needs to have these attributes in some degree to form rehabilitation relationships with members. No one has all these qualities to the degree Thresholds would like, and people are encouraged to motivate themselves or to seek supervisory help to develop attributes that they have the least of and to strengthen the areas that are nascent. Once in a while, all of us will come across a "natural," a person who exemplifies most of these attributes to a startling degree without apparent effort. That might be in one out of a hundred staff. Yet the rest of us share a fair number of these characteristics, too. If you did not share them, for example, you would not be reading this volume. Underdogitis is a "do-gooder" attitude that is a blessing, and we've all got a piece of it. Embracing that part of oneself that wants to leave the world just a little bit better touches a deep need of many staff. This is more than "just a job."

At the same time, we must realize that the rehabilitation relationship has within it the potential for great power over others. It is hard to believe that many psychiatric rehabilitation staff misuse that power to any significant degree, but once aware of the possibility, we need to be mindful of avoiding the mere exercise of power without the healing of a rehabilitation relationship. As has been eloquently stated,

> When we make the transition to being a professional clinician, our culture and human service institutions grant us a broad range of power over the lives of people who are in distress. With that power comes enormous responsibility and great risk. Our responsibility is to never lose sight of the fundamental sanctity, dignity and sovereignty of another human being no matter what their diagnosis may be, no matter how "regressed" or "poor" their prognosis may be, and no matter what their disability may be. The risk is that the power which is granted and which we also assume as clinicians, can begin to eat away at our values and ideals such that we fail to safeguard and uphold the fundamental sanctity, dignity and sovereignty of those whom we seek to serve. The danger is that we can over identify with the professional roles we play and forget the people we are. The danger is that our minds can become severed from our hearts such that our human hearts no longer guide, inform, and shape our work with people. [Deegan, 1990, p. 303]

Having taken an overview of the staff qualities that create the rehabilitation relationship, we can now look more closely at some specific relationship factors and examples of their application.

Empathy, Hope, Trust, and Attachment in the Rehabilitation Relationship

Just because staff have reached out to a person with neurotransmitter/stress syndrome, as we prefer to call "mental illness," in a relationship with all the qualities just described and in the practical programs described in Chapter Four, it does not follow that this is all that requires staff attention. The human condition is such that we all are prone to "neurotic" states that have a direct relationship to parental upbringing; psychological defects; health and birth trauma; guilt; and/or nonsupportive, nongiving, or nonexistent relationships. In short, some bad things happen in everyone's life, whether he or she is mentally ill or not, schizophrenic or not. We need to be aware that such bad things exist in the lives of our members in addition to their illness. For instance, we need to think and feel empathically about the self-hate and deep disappointment that the illness brings up in our members. These are psychological issues with which members need help that we can provide, although currently, all too often, our programs do not allow this help to be offered in a direct way.

We need to provide greater access to specialized psychotherapy services for our members who can use them. Probably the majority of our members do not have the attributes necessary to benefit from traditional psychotherapy, but they all can use individualized psychological support. We need to put our own spin on the ball and translate traditional clinical therapy into our own brand of support, our own rehabilitation relationship therapy.

Almost all members can use rehabilitation relationship therapy. It occurs when the staff-member relationship is enriched by the willingness of staff to take on members' pragmatic needs and to manifest the other personal attributes described here, and the result makes for a powerful and healing combination for many members. Many psychiatric rehabilitation or clubhouse agencies deliberately do not make rehabilitation relationship therapy available, but at Thresholds, it is there for those members who are able to make use of it.

The line between doing what is pragmatic and rehabilitation relationship therapy is murky and sometimes nonexistent. Pragmatic activity is definitely psychotherapeutic, and frequently the psychotherapeutic side carries over into the pragmatic. For instance, when we help members through a program component (a pragmatic step) and they find and acknowledge the strength they have within themselves (as a result of the rehabilitative relationship), that is a wonderful combination. Our strength becomes theirs.

In this rehabilitation relationship, each staff person needs to be the person that he or she is, first and foremost. He or she must reach out from his or her own personhood and connect with each member's personhood. The connection cannot take place between a "professional" and a "patient." We use our professional expertise to guide and teach members, but we connect from our personhood to their personhood.

The most valuable thing we can do for our members within the connection established by the rehabilitation relationship is to impart hope to them. Hope can engender within them the will to live, can open them to new and effective ways of learning, and can lead them to a sense of achievement and self-pride. Hope can best be imparted to another through relationship, through intimacy. The old concepts governing therapy and professionalism—the blank persona, the maintaining of detachment, and so on—will not work with our members given their intensity of fear, deprivation, and loss of hope. Staff must maintain hope and show it freely and visibly to members. They must see each member as an individual so that they can always maintain hope for that person, no matter what has happened in the member's relationships with others. That is a distinguishing feature of the rehabilitation relationship, its capacity to impart hope, dispel apprehension, and nurture the belief that the future beckons with the promise of change.

We are not going to be able to reweave the tapestries of members' lives (their illness, their prior experiences, their personalities), but we can hope to alter enough of the threads to affect the tapestry in some positive manner. Every moment of union with others enriches the tapestry of our lives. Some moments enhance the interior; others embellish the border. All shape the design.

Now, this moment, is all that we have. Our lives, our therapies, our relationships are made up of moments, and so we need to make each moment count. Moments are what are remembered, yet we cannot chose which moments will have an impact on members or be remembered. Therefore, we need to make the most of as many moments as we can, although without berating ourselves for the moments we miss. Those missed moments can be great learning experiences for us and, thus, can let us make more of the next opportunity that arises. When we make a mistake, it can also be a great opportunity for us to admit our error to a member. Such admittance speaks to our basic humanness and can lead to our greater intimacy with members. At times, such a staff admission can be *the* moment of importance for a member.

In making many moments count, the concept of bearing witness applies. Just "being there" for the long haul—bearing witness to the struggle members must undergo and letting them know we are there, we are caring, we will stay even if we cannot substantially change what they are going through—is very important. Bearing witness offers credibility to their pain. It does not leave them alone.

Trust is essential in forming the rehabilitation relationship. Trust leads to the feeling of safety and of being protected. Members need that feeling before they begin to move toward growth, which in its very nature is risk taking. Giving members a way of making sense of their world, their thoughts, and their symptoms, of reframing them in a manner that works, is an achievable art. Members who gain a sense of order and predictability in their lives, can begin to have lives that feel normal and comfortable. Order bespeaks purpose, and purpose can put members within a framework of normalcy. To offer members our integrity is to offer them a sense of their own worthiness, to offer them respect, to treat their lives and their personhood with dignity, and to let them know they deserve all this merely by their very being.

Trust means "confidence in integrity, ability, character, and truth of a person or thing" (*Oxford Dictionary,* 8th ed.) However, the inner feeling engendered by trust does not become manifest in that dictionary definition. To trust staff, a member must go through a process whose exact nature is almost indefinable but that is characterized by what staff do to earn trust.

First and foremost, staff must deliver the goods: that is, they must not make promises they are not going to keep. To the homeless, the promise may just be "I'll come back here tomorrow to see how you are." To the new member, it may be "I'll spend time on crew with you each day until you are settled in." Our willingness to meet the member on his or her own grounds, to listen and offer support, to be there and to care is the foundation upon which trust is built. Trust, like a pearl, starts as just a small grain of something new. It builds from the confidence members develop in their relationships with staff. This is a demanding process that must be met with all the integrity, ability, character, and truth we can muster. By the time a member reaches our agency, the system and the professionals within it may have failed that member time and time again. The mere fact that many agencies must have a homeless program speaks volumes to the failures of the system and the challenge that we face in building trust.

As trust is developing so is the understanding that can be characterized as a *rehabilitation agreement,* and the two commingle. A rehabilitation agreement begins with a member's expectations about the agency. It is our obligation to know these expectations, because if we do not, we will fail our mission in the member's eyes and lose any trust we have achieved. This is not to say that we must agree to all member expectations, but we do have a responsibility to learn what is expected of us and to negotiate those expectations into a reasonable, mutually agreeable framework.

The rehabilitation agreement and trust build upon one another. The agreement does not spring into existence merely because someone asks for a service we offer. It grows just as trust grows. And the fact that its details must be spelled out cannot be overemphasized. No step can be too small. The danger lies in the expectation of member progress in steps that are too big. Small, clearly defined steps allow for much-needed recognition. Small clearly defined steps also enhance communication. Because of the very nature of severe and persistent mental illness, we must invest significant energies communicating clearly, concretely, and empathically with members. If the rehabilitation agreement is obfuscated by unreachable goals, or vague promises, or lack of staff participation, it is doomed to failure.

One of the chapter authors, Jay Forman, remembers teaching his children how to ride their first bicycle:

> At first, they wanted little to do with the process. The training wheels offered all the support they needed. As they rode more and more, the training wheels became more and more of a hinderance. We did not remove the training wheels at first; we just kept raising them farther and farther off the ground. Eventually, we got to the point where the wheels had to come off, and I had to run alongside. Squeals of "don't let go, don't let go" still bring a smile to my face. There was a lot of trust in those three words. But I could only run so far, so often, and so much. Soon, I had to let go.

The relationship and the milieu, like training wheels, can carry members a long way. However, staff cannot fulfill all the obligations of the rehabilitation agreement anymore than training wheels can really teach children to ride bicycles. At some point, the children have to agree to take some risks. Taking risks means being able to trust someone, even if that someone is yourself.

Risk taking begins very early in the rehabilitation process and is also commingled with the development of trust. In fact, risk taking that falls short of the stated goal may be the most important aspect of trust evolution. The member who tries and falls short but who is held in high esteem for trying enhances his or her relationship with the rehabilitation professional. It is never the effort to succeed that hurts people but how that effort is perceived. If people lose self-esteem as a result of trying and falling short, they will stop trying.

Risks are the seeds of empowerment. Small risks followed by praise, supported with empathy, nurtured by understanding will give rise to ever larger efforts on the part of the member. But don't let go, at least not yet. First, staff have to run alongside. This may mean assisting members in going on interviews, cleaning a room or a house, finding a new residence, maintaining physical health, using leisure time, maintaining family relationships, developing a social life, and learning how to seek and hold a job, in addition to being members' advocate for social security income (SSI and SSDI), making absolutely sure the member does not slip through the cracks of the wider mental health and support systems, and engaging in a thousand other efforts. At Thresholds, necessary staff assistance can also include helping a member to shower; delousing a member (a very unpleasant task but sometimes absolutely necessary before an emergency room will serve a member); shopping with or for the member for food or clothes; doing laundry with or for a member; driving a member to a doctor or clinic appointment and waiting with the member until its completion; making sure the member gets food stamps, a rent subsidy, or a clothing allowance; and helping a member manage his or her money so it lasts the entire month, while encouraging the member's own management ability (Thresholds is the representative payee for more than four hundred of its members.) Such mundane but crucial and pragmatic tasks are the backbone of a rehabilitative program. After all, if we do not do it, it does not get done and causes a member either to experience severe neglect or to spin out into a regressive cycle that more often than not leads to hospitalization.

Every goal in the rehabilitation contract deserves the same effort. There is a lot to be accomplished. At the outset, what is most important to the member is the fact that *we* (the member and a staff person) can do it together—just don't let go! Glickman (1992) has said it well: "People don't get better or stronger because someone moves away from them. They get stronger because someone . . . knows them and respects them and needs their help and talents and seeks them out on a regular basis, and therefore what we must do as staff is invest anything we think is good for the members with enormous passion of our own" (p. 55).

The way staff actions and expectations influence member behavior are illustrated by a story chapter author Diane Farrell tells about an agency camping trip:

> Two young men wandered off one evening. A third person in the Young Adult Program told us one of them had marijuana in his tent and even showed it to us. When the first two came back, we accused them of smoking pot, but they would not admit it. It was determined that the one who brought it would be sent back to Chicago and the other allowed to stay. I was the caseworker for the one who stayed, and knowing the other kid would never tell on him, I asked him to tell me the truth about whether or not he had smoked it or not. I told him that what he said would affect how I felt about him. He then told me he had smoked pot on the walk. Later that evening, he told me he had never in his life told the truth when he was in such a situation. He added that no one had ever said it

would really matter what he said and that it was my saying it mattered that had made the difference. I believe the thread of intimacy between us allowed him to tell the truth.

Farrell also recalls a series of meetings with a member who was a survivor of incest that show how the rehabilitation relationship grows:

> Each session was done at her group home rather than the agency and lasted for several hours. During the sessions, she hugged her childhood teddy bear and discussed how vital it was to her during the incest. The mouth had been ripped off (by her as a child, because she was not supposed to tell), and the bear was quite old and tattered now. After our third or fourth session (many sessions involved hugging and comforting), I suggested that perhaps she did not need this bear anymore. She agreed, but we both knew she needed a substitute. We went to several stores together, and finally she saw a bear she wanted. I bought it but said she could have only one bear at a time; the other needed to be in my office. Recently, during my absence because of illness, this member put my perfume on the "new" bear to remind her of me! This intimacy we established was definitely part of a rehabilitation relationship.

The use of touch can be very important in establishing and maintaining the rehabilitation relationship. Hugging, pats on the back, holding a hand in a comforting manner are all very much a part of the rehabilitation relationship. Of course, it is vital to determine how the member feels about touch and to respect that feeling. Some members will definitely not feel comfortable about being touched. Others will absolutely need touch as part of the healing process of growth. It would be sad to deprive those in need of a human loving touch. Farrell and a sexually abused and neglected young woman have used the terms "heart daughter" and "heart mother" in their sessions to describe their relationship. "It is my love and my hope that helps her to hang on," says Farrell, "and it is important for me to be able to say, 'I love you,' and I do. She told me she had to wait for nineteen years for the love she never had, but it was worth it!"

It is all right, even necessary, to foster dependency at the beginning of the rehabilitation relationship. Staff need to do that to forge the bond, to establish trust, to begin intimacy, to begin the process of building a framework that members can buy into, live with, and grow within. Later, members will have more and be more, and then they can move toward independence. But staff cannot expect them to be independent when they do not feel they have any framework of support.

Staff need to use the rehabilitation relationship constructively. Many members will indicate that they can deal with staff anger but not staff disappointment. Thus, it is all right to be angry with members' behavior but not to be punitive and not to hold on to the anger. It is important both to set limits (perhaps the most important way to show one cares) and to nurture. It is also important to know how and when to do each. We are usually told not to "lead" in therapy, but it can be very helpful to offer options or explanations if we can do so as part of building a framework for members and without cramming them down members' throats. The rule is that we should let go right away if the member does not accept a suggestion.

We need to look at the nature of our relationships with each other as well as our relationships with members to understand the nature of the rehabilitation relationship. Do we allow ourselves to love each other? Or is love not an acceptable therapeutic "technique"? At Thresholds, staff believe it is the humanness within each of us that is the primary determinant of the worker we may be able to become.

Recently a staff member who was considered extremely effective left Thresholds, and it is instructive to attend to what members said to him when he said his goodbyes to them during their weekly community meeting: "you listened to me"; "you never yelled at me" (although he did at times!); "you taught me lots when playing ball with me"; "you accepted me"; "you validated me." Interestingly, all these comments reflected interactions that the caseworker had with members within the community milieu rather than the individual session.

Another way to view relationships that can heal and promote growth is through the concept of *attachment*. Attachment is an affectional and emotional bond. It is by definition selective and exclusive. Thus, it cannot be interchanged. Typically, members attach to staff who they feel value them and hold them out as special. Often, residential workers and workers within the rehabilitation milieu are particularly able to establish attachment. As they provide members with special activities and interact informally, they have numerous opportunities to send the message "you are special." Attachment is best nurtured by concrete interactions involving normalizing experiences. In nurturing and setting limits, it is important for the same person to do both because a member will only accept the limits from people with whom he or she feels some sense of attachment.

The sense of security and safety that fosters exploration and growth is developed through a long association based on attachment. The more secure members feel within the attachment relationship, the more they will be able to venture outside to explore and practice new behaviors and relationships. The more secure a member is in one attachment relationship, the more likely it is that he or she will form additional attachment relationships. Moreover, when a member has a primary attachment relationship with one staff person, it is imperative that other staff work collaboratively with that staff person.

When we understand the importance of these attachment principles, we can easily see how a member may attach to various staff members: to crew leaders who can recognize and praise a member's strengths, to group leaders who listen at just the right time, to residential staff who always have time for that "casual" walk around the block.

A former Thresholds member who has since become a staff person had this to say about what creates the attachment in rehabilitative relationships: "I have had numerous psychiatrists and therapists. I was never able to form a bond with them. Thresholds offers love and caring. Both are very much needed. But I can't imagine what Thresholds would be without faith and hope. It is offered because it is genuine and the member can't succeed without it."

In the recent book *The Quiet Room,* one of the authors describes reporting to her psychiatrist that her voices are telling her not to trust him (Schiller and Bennett, 1994). The psychiatrist offers her a reasonable, probably correct but clearly intellectual explanation of auditory hallucinations. Her immediate response was to feel he was completely unable to relate to her and thus unable to help her at all. A person practicing rehabilitation relationship therapy would have seen the need for an empathic response to reflect the client's fear and would have tried to elicit from her a way in which he or she might provide some safety. Interpretations and instructional replies would only come way down the road.

Another example of working on attachment before making suggestions and setting limits involves a member of the Thresholds Young Adult Program who came to his caseworker's office very distraught and angry, complaining about his teachers. He had left the classroom and was refusing to return. The caseworker listened (the number one skill required in a rehabilitation relationship) as he unleashed a torrent of complaints and problems, too many to handle in the few minutes they would have together to work on this. Her goal became to make him feel heard and to offer some hope of working out at least a small part of the problem. Thus, they worked together on "listing" what was going on and on what she might be able to do to help him handle some of the problems. There could be no global resolution at this point, but as the member calmed down, he said a very interesting thing. He knew that the caseworker had been undergoing chemotherapy treatments for some time, and as he felt listened to, felt some safety, felt some hope, his comment, seemingly out of the blue was: "That chemotherapy is going to work for you, I know it will." The evocation of this kind of feeling lets us know a rehabilitation relationship is growing. Even when we are attempting to control inappropriate behavior, it is important that the member know that he or she has been listened to. Then the member is much more likely to try techniques to control the behavior. It simply does not work to insist on behavioral change without having an empathic realization of how the member is feeling.

The rehabilitation relationship is the context in which all other components of psychiatric rehabilitation are rendered effective. The rehabilitation relationship is what engages the member and maintains connection. When a member feels safe within a rehabilitation relationship, he or she can benefit from the rest of the agency program. When a member feels cared about and valued as a person he or she is more able to risk trying new things and new behaviors (Horowitz, 1991).

References

Deegan, P. E. "Spirit Breaking: When the Helping Professions Hurt." *The Humanistic Psychologist*, 1990, *18* (3), 301–313.

Glickman, M. "What If Nobody Wants to Make Lunch? Bottom Line Responsibility in the Clubhouse." *Psychosocial Rehabilitation Journal*, 1992, *16* (2), 55–59.

Horowitz, R. "Reflections on the Casework Relationship: Beyond Empiricism." *Health and Social Work*, 1991, *16* (3), 170–175.

Schiller, L., and Bennett, A. *The Quiet Room.* New York: Warner Books, 1994.

RICHARD HOROWITZ is a former staff worker in the Loren Juhl Young Adult Program at Thresholds.

DIANE FARRELL is program director of the Loren Juhl Young Adult Program at Thresholds.

JAY FORMAN is associate director of Thresholds.

JERRY DINCIN is executive director of Thresholds.

Six goals guide the organization and implementation
of a basic program of psychiatric rehabilitation.

Core Programs in the Thresholds Approach

Jerry Dincin

Psychiatric rehabilitation at Thresholds is guided by six goals. These goals form the basis for our service plans, our outlines of a general treatment strategy for each member. Much as the markings on the closet wall at Thresholds' original location marked physical growth, the degree to which a member fulfills the six goals marks his or her progress and growth. Our research department can follow this progress, and we can adjust our programming accordingly.

Thresholds' six goals are as follows:

1. Prevent unnecessary psychiatric hospitalization.
2. Obtain paid employment for every member capable of working.
3. Provide a wide array of housing consistent with member needs.
4. Improve social relationships and communication skills.
5. Offer educational opportunities at the appropriate level.
6. Promote and monitor physical health.

We certainly did not arrive at our six goals by organizing a think tank to contemplate a theoretical framework for doing psychiatric rehabilitation. We never operate that way. Instead, the six goals emerged from members' needs. They demanded our attention. Members throughout the history of Thresholds have striven to remain outside of the hospital, hold down a job, gain an education, find their own housing, and handle stressed-out family situations and shattered social networks. The goal of promoting and monitoring physical health was not as obvious initially, and we did not state it until 1987. But physical health is just as important to the members' quality of life and rehabilitation as the first five goals, and it is a goal we should have been paying more attention to a long time ago.

Because the goals grew from our concerns about the practical and imme-diate needs of the members, they reflect basic values about the quality of life: just about everyone wants a healthy life with friends, a job, an education, and a decent place to live. But besides being worthy in this obvious sense, the six goals are standards against which we can chronicle the successes and short-comings of our program and measure agency achievement. This evaluation component differentiates Thresholds from many other programs with vague outcome criteria—or none at all. Our commitment to evaluation on our six goals has allowed us to prove in concrete terms to ourselves, the outside world, our members, the board of directors, and funding sources that what we do is valuable.

Almost everything we do fits under the rubric of the six goals and results in an overall goal, which is to embrace our members in a comprehensive hug that fosters a new life. The remainder of this chapter examines each goal in turn.

First Goal: Prevent Unnecessary Psychiatric Hospitalization

As described in Chapter One, Thresholds began as a rehabilitation center to help psychiatric patients cross over from a life in the wards of psychiatric hos-pitals to life in the community. Making that transition to a permanent life in the community remains central to our programming today. Thus, it only makes sense that preventing unnecessary hospitalization of members is our and our members' overarching first goal, and that is where Thresholds staff focus much of their energies. Most people, most of the time, do better in the community than in the hospital. I never attached much value to the experience of psychi-atric hospitalization beyond the very important reason of reduction of symp-toms. Certainly, little therapy is accomplished in the relatively short hospital stays of today. The basic resolution of members' issues must come in the cru-cible of life in the community.

Rehospitalizations can be prevented by developing a trusting rehabilita-tion relationship, taking care of seemingly small day-to-day details before they escalate into crises, anticipating emergencies, monitoring member stress, and paying attention to medication compliance. No problem is too small to war-rant staff attention. Frequently, issues staff might think insignificant turn out to be psychologically unnerving to members. Seemingly insignificant activi-ties of daily living cause some of the most troublesome preludes to a hospi-talization, but these issues are generally preventable through the kind of rehabilitation relationship described in Chapter Three. Staff must feel some of the same pain a member feels to present appropriate empathic and thera-peutic options.

By 1976, we became acutely aware that some people were cycling through all the agencies in our region. Every agency knew them. Despite our focus on our first goal, it seemed impossible to find a way to prevent their hospitalization and keep them in the community. They defied all our best efforts at involvement in established programs. We felt a sense of failure and guilt, impotence and frustration. We blamed them and castigated ourselves. We had heard of the PACT program in Madison, Wisconsin, and its new approach demonstrated and evaluated by Leonard Stein and Mary Ann Test (1985) and decided to visit. A two-day sojourn in Madison led to a monumental change at Thresholds. The development of the programs we call Bridge programs were based on the PACT approach, which included a team model with no individual caseloads; home visiting only, no office visits; an assertive style of outreach that would not take no for an answer; and a focus on money management, housing, and medication. We put our own spin on the model by limiting membership in our Bridge program to the most frequent users of the state hospital, those who had a minimum of five psychiatric hospitalizations in their lifetime, three hospitalizations in the prior year, or ninety days of continuous hospitalization. Our concentration and final evaluation criterion was to keep these members out of the hospital. That was and still is the basic goal in Bridge programs, although in recent years we have begun the process of adding other rehabilitation opportunities. Simply put, that goal is stop the revolving door. Do what one needs to do to keep members from returning to the state psychiatric hospital (Witheridge and Dincin, 1985).

In 1978, with the help of Larry Appleby of the Illinois Department of Mental Health (DMH), Thresholds received the first Bridge program grant through the Hospital Improvement Program of the National Institute of Mental Health, a $100,000-a-year grant for three years to demonstrate a reduction in hospitalization days for the fifty persons who returned to the state hospital most often. It was to be a program for members who had been unwilling or unable to use existing programs of area agencies. Prospects for success were considered marginal, but we were optimistic. After the program's shaky start, Tom Witheridge took over the leadership in 1979, and the program's effect began to be felt. We took on the most difficult people, and with our focus on the nitty-gritty details of daily existence, we were able to reduce rehospitalization precipitously. Our first fifty patients had accumulated 3,752 hospital bed–days in the single year prior to entering our program. By the end of their first program year, they had reduced their hospital days by over half, to 1,731. There was a similar drop in the number of hospital admissions (see Chapter Six). Measurable program success showed enormous gains could be made with a home-visiting and practical focus approach that emphasized assertive medication compliance, representative payeeship for effective money management, and maintenance of housing of members.

After these results, DMH picked up the funding for the original grant, and further expansion was inevitable. There are now six Bridge unit locations, including a mobile unit for homeless mentally ill persons, although all Bridge efforts are in vivo, that is, based on reaching out to members where they live, not on a specific program location. In contrast, day programs are based in a building in the community, and members are expected to come to the program site for psychiatric rehabilitation. Like day programs, Bridge programs, also called assertive community treatment (ACT) programs, utilize the six goals of Thresholds, but the emphasis on specific goals varies considerably between programs. All the Bridge units have grown significantly since their inception, almost entirely from state DMH funds plus a City of Chicago project (Witheridge and Dincin, 1985). Taken together, the projects account for a budget of $5,224,000.

While the proven effectiveness of this approach encouraged DMH to fund nine new programs throughout Illinois replicating this model, of which Thresholds received two expansions, unfortunately several of the newly funded agencies are degrading the model by leaving crucial components out of the mix of services. Strong administrative support, positive staff attitude, and the mutual determination to keep members in the community, if at all possible, are important factors that must be present.

I have already stated that medication compliance, money management, and maintenance of housing are crucial. A focus on these three essential issues, along with the fourth issue of substance abuse, accounts for the vast majority of the success of this program.

Medication compliance. Staff use any and all methods to convince members to take their medication. They will fill prescriptions, deliver the medications daily, watch members take medication, and in general be as persuasive as possible in this area.

Money management. A large subgroup of these symptomatic recidivist members do not handle their meager monthly SSI/SSDI checks wisely so that their essentials are paid for and so that the money lasts all month, which is the object of the money management program. Thresholds is representative payee for about four hundred members, a major fiduciary responsibility. Our payee-ship is an absolute necessity for some members whose judgment and impulse control are impaired or whose mental capacity or residual symptoms preclude the responsible handling of money. Staff make every effort to teach members to handle their money, by gradually stretching out the times at which members receive money, from daily money delivery, to twice weekly, to weekly, to twice monthly. Some members learn; others cannot or will not and are appreciative of staff help. Yet others hate it and demand control of their own funds, and naturally, they get it.

Maintenance of housing. Too many members "forget" to pay their rent immediately after receiving their checks, and they spend the money on discretionary items like cigarettes, clothing, drugs, or even a stereo. Other members' symptoms cause disruption in the buildings where they live. Members can and do get thrown out when this happens, and without a roof over their heads, they say the "magic words" at the state hospital and get admitted until the next check arrives. Much effort must be expended to prevent this, especially in areas such as Chicago, where decent housing for psychiatric patients is a scarce and diminishing resource. In the Bridge programs, we handle this through the representative payee program, which ensures that the rent will be paid. Thresholds also develops friendly relationships with the landlords and, in particular, the desk clerks of SRO (single-room occupancy) buildings it uses, with a promise that if unacceptable behavior occurs our staff can be called at any time of the day or night. This reassurance and its demonstrated availability make a huge difference in residential tenure for our members.

Substance abuse. Few of our Bridge program members are interested in treatment for substance abuse as it clearly involves diminishing the taking of drugs that members use to reduce symptoms, to feel better, or out of habituation. The best staff can do is use the staff-member relationship to persuade members to reduce substance use and to control the money members have available.

Bridge programming reflects nine policies.

Home visiting is the main method of contact. Home visiting allows staff to see firsthand how a member is doing and to deal with problems immediately. Members who have little interest in office appointments or day programs or are too disorganized to keep to a schedule or to maintain involvement with others are well served by exclusive use of the home visit.

Services are restricted to the highest priority recipients. Staff work first with the revolving-door clients, the neediest members, not the members with one or two hospitalizations. The usual Bridge member averages eleven hospitalizations before Thresholds staff ever see him or her.

Reduction of hospital use is the explicit mission. Keeping members out of the hospital, of course, is our reason for being. Naturally, we use hospitals when necessary and see their availability as a crucial resource. However, Bridge members are admitted less frequently and for shorter stays than their prior histories would predict.

The nitty-gritty details of everyday life are given close attention. The concrete survival needs of Bridge members—food, shelter, and clothing—must be met first. This activity is foremost in the prevention of hospitalization.

A total team approach is employed. No staff member has a specific caseload; all members are visited on a rotating basis by all the staff, thus reducing staff burnout and providing respite from extremely difficult members or situations in which the chemistry between member and staff just does not work. The staff-to-member ratio is one to ten. This ratio is necessary for this approach to be effective; significant deviation will absolutely lead to the erosion of success. It helps to have a psychiatrist willing to make occasional home visits.

Teams are willing to become the single point of responsibility. The team becomes each member's watchdog, no matter what the problem or where it might occur. This can mean following a member through a jail term or an extensive stay in a state hospital or substance abuse rehabilitation center.

Potential crises are anticipated and prevented. A significant number of hospitalizations are not directly related to symptoms but to member reactions to what seem to members to be insurmountable problems in everyday life. Staff are there to defuse and reframe these problems and to support members at this time.

Staff are easily accessible in times of crisis. During working hours, staff are available on a "drop everything" basis; during nonworking hours, on an on-call basis.

Membership is on a "no-close" basis. Membership in the Bridge program is based on long-term need, not on performance. Members are not closed, or dropped, except when they insist or sometimes when they exhibit dangerous behavior.

The Thresholds Bridge programs have always been successful in reducing hospital days among members because of their adherence to the practice and principles I have described here, coupled with staff determination and spirit. The Bridge programs also confirm a Thresholds pattern: forget theories and do whatever is necessary for any group of psychiatric patients. Our work is focused on the broad group of people with severe and persistent mental illness, not just those who can conform to the clubhouse model.

Good work sometimes gets rewarded, and Thresholds Bridge won the Frances J. Gerty Award in 1982 from the Illinois Department of Mental Health. In 1981, *Hospital and Community Psychiatry,* the journal of the American Psychiatric Association, bestowed the Significant Achievement Certificate on Thresholds Bridge.

Second Goal: Obtain Paid Employment for Every Member Capable of Working

Most members come to the Thresholds day program with a stated desire to work. Whether that desire matches their capability is unknown at the start, but our belief is that most members truly motivated for paid work can do so, and it is our job to help members realize the goal. This belief is based on a deep respect for the value of work in improving self-image, in gaining self-respect and respect of others, in normalizing the person who works, and for providing an income that produces a number of benefits. It is always wonderful to work and earn money. These are basic notions that are woven into the American cultural pattern and ethos in a deeply meaningful way. Thus, the value of an agency vocational goal is simply the inherent value of work, as supported by our Western culture.

In America, it is better to work than not to work, and it has been my experience that a lot more agency members can work than do. Some members will not succeed at paid work, and Thresholds works just as hard to help them find a pattern of meaningful activity as it does to help others find a job. But we believe that everyone deserves a chance to work, and we give members our best shot at assisting them in this job process. And a process it is, although we are not wedded to any one method of making vocational placements. We utilize supported group employment, transitional employment, long-term individual placements, sheltered workshops, volunteer placements, and members' own jobs. All are legitimate as long as they help members find work. In this field, too much attention is paid to job placement names: for instance, Transitional Employment Program, Supported Job Placement, or Choose-Get-Keep. What really matters is helping members get back to work, not what we call that work. Let's keep our eye on the goal and let the rhetoric be secondary.

The vocational component of Thresholds programming began in 1962 with the introduction of prevocational work crews. The crew system is based on the early Fountain House model in which members volunteer for a work-readiness experience in maintenance, kitchen, or clerical areas. This experience is the prevocational program foundation. Crews provide a structured program in which members improve their work habits and work personality, learning to show up on time, work fast enough and steadily, get along with co-workers and the boss, follow instructions, and show motivation and initiative (Bond and Dincin, 1986). All these factors are evaluated by staff, who work right alongside members on the crew. A combined evaluation by member and staff determines the member's readiness for paid work. Computerized tests, paper-and-pencil exams, or work sample approaches have not proved as valuable for us as the situational assessment that work crews provide (see Chapter Six).

In the early years, we found employers willing to hire our members and then found members willing to do that work on job placements. This method still forms the bulk of vocational opportunities at Thresholds. In addition, we use the current Choose-Get-Keep style of vocational determination. The latter is sometimes plagued by unrealistic job desires while the former is faulted with job mismatching. For many members, a step-by-step job improvement approach offers them the opportunity to improve their job skills at each subsequent job opportunity. However, staff must be careful not to foreclose members' job futures by not offering increasingly challenging jobs. This is another area in which philosophical approach gives way to practical considerations. The most important goal is to get as many members to work as possible, using whatever approach is feasible, in as good a job as each member can hold.

In 1963, when jobs for psychiatric patients were a novelty whose feasibility had not been demonstrated, employers provided only the job opportunity; wages of Thresholds members were paid by a federal grant. But as members' success as workers became evident, employers began to give members carfare, lunch money, and a few dollars. Some of these jobs turned into permanent jobs. Soon after, of course, employers paid the going wage.

In June 1984, 122 members at Thresholds had jobs on 20 Thresholds placements, and 79 had their own jobs. Their projected gross wages for that year were $991,000. Ten years later, in 1994, the number of members working for pay had increased to 414, the number of employers had increased to 135, and yearly projected gross wages were $2.8 million. As the following chart (Table 4.1) from our most recent five-year plan suggests, we are convinced that more members could work if we could develop the employment opportunities.

Table 4.1. Thresholds Employment Goals by Type of Employment

Type of Job	Current Members Working (June 1994)	Proposed Members Working (June 1999)
Members' own jobs	103	130
Individual placements	79	130
Group placements	50[a]	90[b]
Thresholds businesses	49	100
Sheltered workshops	133	100
Below minimum wage	120	80
Above minimum wage	13	20
Total members	414	550

[a] In eight placements.
[b] In twelve placements.

I also think we could shorten the time each member spends in our work-readiness program if more of the right kind of jobs were available for members, although we do have a group of members who need to stay in the work-readiness program for an extended period of time. This is in contrast to the earlier years of the agency, when virtually everyone who came through the doors would be headed toward a job rather quickly. Members enter Thresholds with greater levels of impairment in recent years, and they require more time to go through the work-readiness program.

Group placements. Group placements are my favorite because they employ members in integrated settings with nondisabled co-workers, doing a real job. On group placements, members can lean on the support of other members as well as the job coach. It provides an ideal first step after the work-readiness program.

Current group placements at Thresholds include delivering a weekly newspaper, doing janitorial office cleaning, providing maid service at a hotel, bagging in a supermarket, unpacking clothes in a warehouse, and unloading shoes at a major chain retailer. The door-to-door newspaper delivery placement is nearly ideal. It requires a low level of skill and is an intermittent job. The placement with Dominicks, a major Chicago grocery chain, has been tremendously successful, drawing members from all Thresholds branches. Members can join a union if they are successful in this group placement and transfer permanently to a supermarket in their own neighborhood. Over seven years ago, Thresholds joined with several other agencies, through National Industries for the Severely Handicapped (NISH), in a project known as Jan-Tech to bid successfully on a contract for cleaning a federal government building. Members' work performance in this group placement is graded on a strict scale, and members are paid on that basis. The big advantage to this job is that members who work extremely well can make up to $10 per hour plus benefits.

Individual placements. We feel this is an area that needs much more development (as of June 1994, we had seventy members on individual placements). Currently, most of these placements are part-time jobs in regular businesses, but they are not strictly time limited. In some cases, they can become permanent jobs if the fit is right.

Thresholds businesses. Under the auspices of Thresholds Rehabilitation Industries (TRI), a not-for-profit subsidiary of Thresholds, we provide jobs to members in a variety of agency-owned businesses. TRI Services Cleaning provides janitorial jobs to between thirty and fifty members at a variety of levels, including supervisory roles. Most recent contracts have been for the cleaning of state-owned office buildings. Members at one branch clean a rest area on the Interstate. TRI also continues to do some corporate office cleaning.

TRI operates a thriving thrift shop called Bargains Galore, in which an integrated workforce of members and neighborhood people sell donated clothing and other items as well as purchased furniture. The shop has a van that picks up donations and also does small moving jobs. One of our more intriguing enterprises is a rag business, begun five years ago when too much unusable clothing was being stockpiled at the thrift store. Members use a machine to cut the excess clothing up into rags and then bale them. The rags are sold to the State of Illinois. An additional business is Custom Copy, a rapid copy service that reproduces training manuals and packages other supplies for management training classes for IBM. We are investigating several other business opportunities, and it is clear that Thresholds is moving strongly toward this means of supplying jobs.

The businesses are expected to break even without any subsidy. In fiscal 1994, TRI had a surplus of $30,000 on revenues of $1.8 million. That result requires having someone on staff with a strong entrepreneurial bent.

Sheltered workshops. Although there is some current opposition to sheltered workshops, I think they have a place in the array of work for members because some psychiatric patients, by reason of symptoms or personal habits, cannot work in business or industry without an enormous amount of support. The sheltered workshop is also the right transition step to a first placement, and it is right for people who have not been successful in other placements or who need a respite from stressful placements. However, we have put a cap on the number of people in workshops, and are trying to make sure that every effort is made to move members out into community jobs.

Disincentive to paid work. To do as well as he or she does with SSI, including medical and medication benefits, a member needs to make $15,000 a year. Most members are not capable of working on a full-time basis in order to earn that salary. Indeed, if they earn over $500 a month, their Social Security benefits are reduced, and their medical benefits may be reduced or even discontinued. If a member then has a symptomatic regression, he or she has difficulty getting back on Social Security. For someone who depends on medication to maintain mental stability, this can be a devastating loss, and many members who have a historical pattern of symptom swings prefer not to take the chance of losing benefits. This situation is the single biggest deterrent to getting members back into the workplace.

Volunteer placements. We have never been terribly successful in getting volunteer placements for members. Theoretically, volunteer placements would be great for certain members. A volunteer placement can engender a sense of usefulness in a member and a feeling of contributing to society. Currently, we have some members with over five years of continual work in a volunteer capacity. We need to start emphasizing volunteer placements to a greater degree.

In brief, our experience at Thresholds suggests these guidelines for a vocational program:

Moving toward a paying job is a central piece of the psychiatric rehabilitation of most members.

All methods of job placement should be fully utilized.

Sheltered workshops are necessary but should be used sparingly and with intelligence and sensitivity, always with an eye to movement toward community jobs.

Agency businesses are a good idea and can be break-even propositions. Agencies are limited here only by their own creativity.

Work-readiness programs are an important and usually necessary prevocational evaluation experience. They help members become both more confident and job ready and help staff knowledgeably assist members in overcoming deficits hindering their progress.

In the awful rush to "medicalize" all agency services so they will be supported by Medicaid, do not forget to fund vocational rehabilitation. It works.

Third Goal: Provide a Wide Array of Housing Consistent with Member Needs

When Thresholds started housing members over twenty years ago, staff were responding to a very basic problem: too many places where members lived were awful, disgraceful, and insulting. They were psychiatric ghettos, disgusting SROs, or miserable apartments or boarding homes. And there were no alternatives. Many members lived with their parents, a situation that has its own set of disadvantages for both member and parent although usually acceptable as housing. Since a decent affordable array did not exist in Chicago in 1970, having our own housing became a prime goal for us. We have progressed from providing 4 beds to 489 beds, and we have a goal of 800 beds by the year 2000. I have never had any doubt that psychiatric rehabilitation should be in this business.

We use a very simple criterion to evaluate whether housing is decent: is it good enough for our own brother or sister? An array of such decent housing is key in our concept, including group homes, clustered and scattered apartments, and entire buildings of studio apartments. (Other valuable types, although not in the Thresholds array, are intermediate care facilities [ICFs], room-and-board houses, Fairweather Lodges, foster homes, and intergenerational housing, and more types will surely be invented [Dincin, 1988]). Each type has its own function and rationale within a comprehensive system.

Group homes. While no single housing style can be right for our varied population, we do have a preference for group homes. Most members need the nurturant living situation that is best exemplified in a group home of high quality. The milieu that can be created in a group home is actually healing for many members. Every psychiatric rehabilitation agency believes in the importance of its overall milieu and the milieu of its day program. Milieu also makes a difference in housing. Group homes offer a sense of belonging in a family-type communal living situation that is frequently also expressed in our culture in the college fraternity or co-op.

There are many positive aspects of small group home living that cannot be easily duplicated in individual apartments: for instance, the availability of a variety of people with whom to try out new friendship and independence skills, of companionship without the necessity of intense intimacy, and of peers when the member does not need professional help but is nevertheless lonely. Many persons with severe and persistent mental illness have had their normal developmental process interrupted by hospitalization or symptom development. Many still need to go through the normal stages in some modified form and at their own pace. Group living can offer them this opportunity.

Group homes can also be a significant help for many special populations. Eighteen- to twenty-two-year-olds usually need a strong structure and limit setting not easily offered to people in scattered apartments. A group home also gives them the opportunity to work on separation issues and to develop effective interpersonal ability with peers and staff. The deaf mentally ill, among other special needs groups, are best accommodated in group homes since their illness itself is so isolative.

Members need peer support, and the friends they develop in mental health settings are frequently the only friends they have. The most lasting and meaningful of these friendships are frequently spawned in group homes, and helping members develop such friendships in their natural peer groups is beneficial because it gives members a crucial sense of warmth and connectedness.

In my opinion, personal growth, particularly after a recent release from a mental hospital, does not occur best when members live in scattered apartments, an arrangement that emphasizes loneliness instead of growth and interaction. Yet growth can not be encouraged for all people in the same way. Clearly there are many people who are basically loners, who cannot stand group living and cannot or will not cooperate in group activities, and there are also those who can and should be living independently. No housing model can be completely rejected, because when well executed each has significant strengths and can be naturally and completely supportive. Members should have a strong say in where they live, but that does not mean staff should not offer alternatives. There definitely are drawbacks to group living for some people; however, it is also true that many people have found great comfort, solace, and growth in group homes and, indeed, have made the transfer of training necessary to become independent and have enjoyed their experiences. As of 1995, Thresholds owned or operated twenty-seven group homes for 241 people.

Supported housing. Supported housing in both clustered and scattered apartments is another good option. However, we should remember that members with substance abuse problems almost always want their own apartments and generally for all the wrong reasons—so they can be alone to use drugs or alcohol. Conversely, complete reliance on supported housing can result in members' overdependence on professional support when members could be turning to peers in times of need or desire for company. Currently, Thresholds operates eight apartment houses for 169 people, and sixty scattered apartments housing 103 people. Although it is theoretically desirable for people with severe and persistent mental illness to integrate their social lives with their neighbors', this is an almost completely unrealistic expectation. Whom are we kidding? For the most part, members are too ill, too symptomatic, and too disabled to move into an independent apartment successfully, even with good support. Thus, supported living in studio apartments, either clustered or scattered, is valuable for the many members for whom group living is too stressful or otherwise inappropriate. For the homeless mentally ill, this is especially true. Apartments in all forms constitute the largest number of our units. Each completely renovated studio unit has its own bathroom, small kitchen, and living room/bedroom.

Supervision. All of Thresholds congregate housing is staffed twenty-four hours a day. For younger or more disturbed populations—mentally ill substance abusers (MISAs), older adolescents, and the hearing impaired—we require awake shift staff; in programs for other groups, staff sleep at night. For the most part, there is no vocational rehabilitation offered at the residences; members come to the day program for the bulk of their rehabilitation. The exceptions are the totally in-house programs for the hearing impaired and our three new MISA group homes (see Chapter Five).

Board involvement. The involvement of an agency's board of directors can be an important asset in a housing program. Our board, for example, has contributed funds to purchase two group homes, and board members have brought their business skills to bear, looking closely at each housing venture in terms of capital planning, renovations, legal issues, and architecture and imparting a strong sense of solid business real-estate development practices. They have helped ensure that we maintain our housing in a good manner, and we now employ a full-time property manager to monitor leases, maintenance, and repairs with the goal of each house being the best maintained house on its block.

Capital funds. Obtaining capital funds for acquisition, construction, and renovation of housing is a crucial problem, and one solution has been to use HUD Section 202 and 811 programs. Through these programs, we have built ten group homes and three apartment houses. We find it takes close to five years from the first submission of a HUD application until the first member moves into the building. A hired consultant facilitates our negotiations with HUD because some of the processes are very technical and arduous, especially in Chicago.

Clearly, every locale needs to find its own source and mix of capital funding. Thresholds, for example, has received capital funds from the Illinois Housing Development Authority, the City of Chicago, several foundations, and its own directors. It has participated in bond funding through the Illinois Health Facilities Authority, but legal and other bond-financing costs make this an unattractive avenue in the future. We are currently working on projects that layer one source of funding on another. Bank mortgages are also available, and we have used Low Income Housing Credits.

Operational funds. The vast majority of operational funds for staff and residential programs are provided by DMH and, to a minor degree, Title XX of the Social Security Act. The Illinois Department of Children and Family Services (DCFS) provides funds for our residential program for older adolescents. Two group homes are self-supporting through fees paid by parents.

Community opposition. Nothing incenses me quite as much as the opposition we have encountered over the years to bringing housing into the community, and there does not seem to be any right or correct way to handle this opposition and the prejudices that lead to the fears community residents have for their safety. What I can report is that once the housing has been occupied for six months, in every single case, the opposition diminishes and then disappears. Sometimes we have formed neighborhood advisory boards, but they soon disband because of the lack of complaints. We just fade into the neighborhood woodwork, but nobody believes in advance that this will happen. Thus, we feel it is usually better to let as few people as possible know of an impending development. Of course, that leaves us open to the charge of "sneaking in," but we find that easier to deal with than the virulent opposition we meet if we publicize our intentions. In the end, time and good experience are the only ways to overcome community resistance toward establishing housing for the mentally ill.

Moreover, we cannot allow community opposition to derail us from delivering a constructive and viable choice in housing to members, en route to creating the best climate for their independence. We must continue to give them a choice in housing, as is their right and a crucial part of their rehabilitative process. The Federal Fair Housing Act is by far our greatest ally here. This law can be an absolute blessing. It is favorable to our members' civil rights and carries such strong penalties that it does not even have to be invoked to be an effective and formidable tool.

A climate for independence. In line with the rest of our aims, we strive to create a climate for separation and independence from parents in member housing, and most people do move from a dependent to a more independent level of housing during their membership at Thresholds. While members' most obvious dependent relationship is with family, members can also become dependent on the daily care provided by nursing homes and ICFs. Breaking member dependence on these care facilities can be achieved as part of the overall rehabilitation process as members gain more confidence in other areas of their lives. Breaking the dependent relationship with the family is trickier. The transition away from the family is difficult enough that Thresholds Parents/Relatives Group spends several sessions on this issue, and questions about separation constantly come up in other meetings with families.

Thresholds has consistently given the message that the greatest love parents can show a child is to allow and encourage him or her to separate from the parental home. We strongly believe that living at home is usually counterproductive in the long term and that psychological damage can result for both parent and child if either is unable to let go. For some parents, this message is quite a shock. They felt they were being models of good parenting by maintaining their mentally ill child at home, even when their effort left them drained emotionally, physically, and financially.

Parents need to see this emancipation as an act of love, not rejection. The member's independence and maturity depend on it. But freeing the child can also reignite old feelings of guilt and despair in parents. Members may manipulate this by asking, "If you love me, why do I have to leave?" Freeing the child must come as an act of love, with parents displaying the boundary-setting attitudes and the presentation of a unified front that they use in other areas of childrearing.

The Parents/Relatives Group wrestles with the question of emancipation in four ways. First, the concept of good parenting is discussed, with stress on the child's independence as a goal. Second, parents face the question of their mortality: how are they preparing their child to live without them when they die? Third, parents confront the idea that *they* will have to mobilize the latent strength of their child to achieve independence if they do not support Thresholds in providing the opportunity, the know-how, and the facilities to help the child become independent. Fourth, parents face the probability that there is little potential for the member's growth in the parental home. Letting go is a hard but essential part of the rehabilitation process.

However difficult it is, I strongly urge psychiatric rehabilitation agencies to get into the housing arena and to deliver an array of housing opportunities. As caring professionals, we owe that quality of life to our members, and I can testify that it is within the reach of psychiatric rehabilitation.

Fourth Goal: Improve Social Relationships and Communication Skills

From the earliest days, when members packed 1153 North Dearborn playing games and holding discussions, to today, when members have a number of Thresholds clubhouses and drop-in centers available, Thresholds has helped members move toward an improved social and recreational life. While this social goal may not have been stated or written down in the early days, it has always held a central position in Thresholds programming.

This goal, too, seems obvious because it is value driven. It is better to have friends and participate in leisure time activities than to isolate oneself and be alone. However, it also is the goal most difficult to meaningfully quantify and analyze, and we have not done as good a job in measuring progress on this goal as I would like.

Mental illness tends to separate members from their earlier peers, their families, and the general population, and the symptoms of mental illness almost always include a diminished capacity to enter into and enjoy social relationships. Therefore, it is a difficult task to help members make changes in their social habits. When suffering with the positive symptoms of schizophrenia or the highs of mania, members are nearly inapproachable and reject contact and input. When experiencing the negative symptoms of schizophrenia or the lows of depression, members have no energy, are apathetic, and feel hopelessness. At both ends of the symptom spectrum, friends and enjoyable social events recede and diminish.

The clubhouse. We have found that the very best environment for combating this result is the clubhouse, a naturalistic setting. Club members do not just sit around in their clubhouse. They are active in one facet of it or another. One of the major socializing components of a clubhouse setting is the work crew. On these crews, members work together and become acclimated to interacting with other people. Members frequently fail on job placements because of their inability to interact acceptably. With the exception of a few job placements, such as some maintenance jobs, members at work must regularly interact with the public, fellow employees, and supervisory personnel. While these interactions may not appear in job descriptions, on-the-job socializing has a paramount place in determining a member's perceived performance, since perceptions of employee job performance are often shaped by social interactions. If a fellow employee or supervisor is asked to judge the work performance of a member who does not interact on the job, at coffee breaks, or at lunch, the evaluation will be tainted by that lack of social interaction. We need each other and feel a loss when no contact with fellow human beings is forthcoming. A red flag appears when a member spends coffee breaks sitting off to the side not speaking with anyone or just listening to the conversation of others. Such odd or different behavior is noticed and commented on by fellow workers. On that level, socialization skills have a very real and practical meaning: they improve the marketability of members in the workplace. In addition, socialization in the workplace can also be therapeutic.

Of course, there are other dimensions to social interactions. There is the pleasure of simply connecting with another human being, the sense of participation in a group activity, and the potential of more intimate relationships. We are, by our very nature, somewhat social beings, and while isolation and separateness are every person's right, at Thresholds, many members are socially inhibited by fear of rejection, self-absorption, personal pain, and other symptoms directly related to their illness. Our job in psychiatric rehabilitation, therefore, is to develop programs and promote an atmosphere that makes it easier and more pleasurable for members to relate to other individuals and groups.

The Thresholds method is to find and emphasize a member's positive attributes then build from there. Staff try to enhance members' social skills in three areas: they help members learn conversational skills, establish and maintain acquaintances and deeper and more intimate relationships, and make more interesting and productive use of their leisure time. Teaching social skills is difficult to do and difficult to measure. Part of the difficulty may be overcome by the force of the social milieu within a clubhouse. The atmosphere and interaction between staff and members, staff and staff, and members and members spawns a natural socialization. At Thresholds, we want to reduce members' sense of isolation and increase their interaction with the community at large. That is one of the reasons we think it is so important to be open on evenings and weekends, so that members have many more opportunities to interact than to isolate themselves.

Members sometimes need to relearn how to have fun; it is a major component of the social experience. Staff, while remembering their professional responsibilities and taking a leadership role, participate as fellow human beings in outings and events. Psychiatric rehabilitation relies on such person-to-person relationships and on respecting members as active participants in their own social recovery.

Additional socialization activities. The Thresholds social program occurs through formal groups as well as through the informal clubhouse socialization. The more formal socialization is experienced via activity groups, conversation groups, and problem-solving groups. Socialization within the milieu stresses the normalization of one-on-one interactions. Members and staff eat together. Coffee breaks are taken as a group during the morning, and much interaction occurs between members. Ordinary questions and discussions about how the Chicago Bears or Bulls or Cubs or White Sox are playing hold a valuable, if perennially frustrating, place in discussion. Staff also address socialization through normal conversational opportunities within the milieu in general, encouraging the casual socialization that occurs in everyday life. It is one of the basic life skills that members need to be taught for the first time or to relearn, rehearse, and utilize.

We also promote socialization, particularly leisure time socialization, through many hours of availability. Our several drop-in centers' greatest value is socialization. The concept is to develop an easy atmosphere with fewer formal groups than the day programs, and each drop-in center tends to develop its own ethos and character. Programming that operates in the evenings and weekends is also very important. Just as important is the programming provided on holidays so that members will not feel a sense of loneliness or isolation aggravated by the holiday spirit of the general population. Thanksgiving Day, Christmas Day, and, to a degree, New Year's Eve are holidays fraught with emotional baggage. We have a duty to provide programming on those days. Holidays such as the Fourth of July, Memorial Day, and Labor Day are important for their place as times for leisure and fun. We also have our own celebrations in the form of the Member Recognition Days described in Chapter Two. In a similar vein, a banquet for working members recognizes the importance of members' employment, giving members a sense of accomplishment. On this occasion, Thresholds also honors the businesses who employ our members. Photos are taken and a meal eaten. Both recognition events are dress-up occasions.

Members have also experienced some very creative social outings. Groups of them have gone apple picking, fishing, horseback riding, golfing, picnicking, and bowling. They have gone together to movies, museums, and several styles of musical events. Free passes are available almost monthly for a buffet and a play at a local theater. On a yearly basis, tickets are available from several professional sports organizations. Sports events tend to be highlights for members. We also encourage expressive arts, to foster both socialization and creativity, through newsletters, our literary magazine (*Musing Place*), art and photography shows, theater productions, craft exhibits, movement groups, and a choral group.

All our efforts at giving our members better social experiences arise from our belief that improved socialization is the foundation on which the lives of our members can be maintained in a meaningful and worthwhile manner outside of the hospital setting.

Possible degree of socialization. Lots of measures exist in the mental health field for measuring socialization, but I am not satisfied that they provide the information we require: Do our members have relationships? Do they use their leisure time well? Do they have a social network? Whether our members have the ability to attain a reasonably high degree of social integration with general society is also an interesting question. It has been our experience that members generally do not integrate to any significant degree with general society. We do not see many of them joining bowling leagues, dart teams, the Elks, or the Moose. Too often, members are just different enough in how they present themselves that they do not integrate well with general society, only with other members and their own families. There are many exceptions, of course. Members do become active in church groups, and members who are not symptomatic for extended periods of time may become involved in other normalized activities.

However, I think we fool ourselves if we think the majority of our severely and persistently ill members are going to integrate fully with the larger society. I am not even sure that the stress of trying to integrate, admirable goal though integration is, is worth the payoff. Of course, a significant group of psychiatric patients do achieve this integration, but these people tend not to need or use our services.

The net result is that Thresholds must create a relatively permanent social setting to combat the withdrawal and isolation endemic to our members. The real and deep loneliness that accompanies the onset of schizophrenia or bipo-lar illness and the resultant severing of ties with former friends and family is very painful. That is why Thresholds finds it essential to make a viable long-term commitment to provide an ongoing social life for its members, and not necessarily with the expectation that members are going to integrate into gen-eral society.

Camping as a model of socialization. The camp experience stamps its mem-ories indelibly on the campers in a way no other part of Thresholds program-ming does. Having fun is a wonderful memory to have and hold, and that is exactly what happens at camp. Nothing at Thresholds better epitomizes the ideal relationship between staff and members or better illustrates the concept of psychiatric rehabilitation than our camping program and the significance of its lasting memories. Members and staff at camp are thrown into a "must" situ-ation, separated from the everyday world and forced to rely on one another and to survive unexpected situations together—as people, not just in their roles as members or staff. Thunderstorms drench a staff person just as thoroughly as a member. Camp erases barriers; people have to develop intimacy. Staff, like members, need to shower, shave, sleep in tents, and use the outdoor rest room.

The camping experience at Thresholds began in the early 1960s at a YMCA camp on the shores of Lake Michigan. In those early years, virtually all the staff and members were out roasting marshmallows, sleeping outdoors, hiking, and living the outdoor life. The usual length of a trip today is five days in summer and a long weekend in winter. Camping trips are more rugged at times, including canoeing trips to Northern Minnesota that can last for nine days, skiing trips to Wisconsin, and backpacking trips to the Porcupine Moun-tains. Thresholds people have also made several rugged excursions with an Outward Bound type of program. On those trips, members tackled the chal-lenges of caving, rock climbing, canoeing, and backpacking.

One staff member noticed that one of two things generally happened upon the members' return from camp. Either members would be so charged up they would want to go on job placement or make some other major changes, or they would be depressed over coming back to the humdrum existence of their daily routines. The stories of members who started to move from their parents' homes or asked to go on a job placement after camping are legion. Camping is a catalyst, but it is also mysterious. What is it exactly that makes it work? We may not understand it, but we feel it. We like to think that members can see what health is like and not be so encumbered by their own difficulties. For many of them, it is a turning point. There is an element of adventure and real spontaneity of fun that they do not see in their everyday lives. Certainly there have been times when members have had difficulties while camping, but those times have been few and far between. The number of times when problems developed from symptomatic members is phenomenally low.

Some of the normalizing and socializing effect is more clearly meaning-ful. Many relationships between campers are cemented over cups of hot chocolate at night, staring into the fire, listening to the crickets and the other surprisingly loud sounds of the woods. Also, a tradition has developed of giving a gift to another camper on the last night of camp. All the members and staff in each camp site exchange names on the first day of camp, and a gift needs to be made for every camper by the end of camp. The gifts may be anything from that special stone polished to glistening by a stream, to a dried flower, to a paperweight made in crafts, and the gift-giving ceremony itself is wrought with meaning. In the end, camp will be remembered more than whether or not a member achieved each goal of his or her service plan on time. The camaraderie will have been cemented on the night a thunderstorm sent everyone scurrying under a shelter roof. It will be remembered even five or ten years later.

Camp is but one of many ways we have responded to special needs that technically fall outside of traditional practice, and that is the Thresholds way: whatever a member needs within the umbrella of our comprehensive approach, we try to provide.

Fifth Goal: Offer Educational Opportunities at the Appropriate Level

Outside light filters through high windows into a classroom at Thresholds Penn House. The room comfortably seats a class of twelve and was one of those fortunate accidents that helped Thresholds grow over the years. A large room in this apartment became available to be turned into a classroom, and it turned out to be perfect for its role. When the class is larger than twelve, the members simply move out into the expansive living room, which is unused during the day. In various ways, we have moved academic education into all our day programs. The fit with our other goals is solid.

Education is important at Thresholds. It is important in itself as it increases the quality of members' knowledge, and it is important practically as it gives members better vocational options. Members are encouraged to go as far as they can or want to in academic pursuits and vocational education. Since the value of education in American society is almost as great as that of work, the normalizing effect of academic achievement is an important motivator for further education. Because schizophrenia often strikes in a person's late teens or early twenties, many members' have had their educational experiences interrupted or ended during high school or college. Some were different from their peers even before the full onslaught of the illness, being depressed, distracted, or symptomatic in the school setting, and the quality of their learning experience suffered. For many members, then, there is a longing to complete what their peers and other family members have completed.

Thresholds breaks education into three primary areas: adult basic education; high school graduation or equivalency; and college-level classes.

Adult basic education. You could call adult basic education reading, writing, and arithmetic. We try to teach these basics at the sixth-grade level to those members who missed them or did not understand them the first time.

High school graduation or equivalency. The high school educational component involves both an accredited high school and a GED program. The Young Adult Program operates the accredited high school, with small classes of six youngsters and highly trained special education teachers. Members earn their high school diplomas, and we hold a meaningful cap-and-gown graduation exercise each year. All these youngsters work hard for their diplomas, and their sense of accomplishment is joyful for them and the audience of parents, peers, and staff.

For adult members, the high school equivalency program is less formal but no less important. Paid teachers and volunteers, some of them members, teach and tutor individuals in the subjects needed to pass the high school equivalency exam. Members derive a great deal of satisfaction from obtaining their GEDs, some going on to college or trade school.

College-level programs. Many members who have had some college would like to complete their education. Others want to start college once they have received their Thresholds high school diplomas but are apprehensive about meeting college academic standards and social expectations. To answer these needs, the Community Scholar Program (CSP) was started at Thresholds in 1988, with demonstration funds from the U.S. Department of Education and two staff. An education coordinator taught classes and provided tutorial assistance. A mobile education worker handled a college support group, on-campus linkage with college teachers, and in-service training at local colleges and vocational schools on mental illness. After the government grant ran out, several foundations stepped in with funding, but keeping this program functioning is a continual struggle, although well worth it.

Since its beginning, the program has served hundreds of members, with 40 percent going on to institutions of higher education or trade schools for further studies. Six members have even gone on to graduate school and one member has completed a doctorate in history. Our research found that the CSP elevated self-esteem and lessened anxiety (see Chapter Six). This is important, since half of those who enter the CSP have a college background, often interrupted by the onset of their illness.

CSP classes include Study Skills, which teaches the basics needed for attending classes: skills in time management, concentration, listening, note taking, test preparation, and test taking as well as vocabulary improvement and memory improvement. In this class, according to the CSP director, "the members blossom from giving a one-minute speech where they are sweaty to giving a five-minute speech like they have done it all their lives." Another class, Research/Writing Skills, guides students through the writing of a research paper: using the library, selecting a topic, formulating a statement of purpose, outlining, selecting references, and collecting data. Interpersonal Communications deals with many areas of verbal and nonverbal communications as they relate to work, school, home, friends, and family. Included are plans for developing appropriate verbal skills for pursuing education: interpreting and understanding nonverbal communication of teachers and classmates, learning the barriers to communication with faculty and other students, building interpersonal communication skills for success, developing oral classroom presentation skills, and cultivating group interaction skills. The tutoring offered in the CSP is provided by staff, peers, and/or tutorial computer programs in reading, language, or math skills. Staff can also link members to tutoring help on campus. The CSP also provides support on an individual basis with staff and in a group setting.

The goal of education excites members in a different way than do the goals of preventing hospitalizations and finding employment. While having the practical side of making a member more employable, education also simply enriches members' lives.

Sixth Goal: Promote and Monitor Physical Health

This goal developed slowly, being added to our list in 1987. The seed was planted through staff attendance at conferences where the physical health needs of psychiatric patients were emphasized. At the time, few psychiatric rehabilitation agencies saw physical health concerns as part of their action mandate. Thresholds realized that for the past thirty years it had left this mandate to others, naïvely believing that someone, somewhere, somehow, was taking care of members' physical health. Belatedly, we saw that this was not happening. For poor people with psychiatric problems, taking care of their own physical health was almost impossible without help. We became determined to offer this help, and gradually, that determination became a full-fledged program goal. We now offer a number of screenings, tests, and activities in the pursuit of members' better health: a yearly physical exam for every member; a yearly SMA-20 blood test for every member; an exercise program at every location, including group homes; an AIDS and STD (sexually transmitted disease) risk assessment; HIV testing, offered for all but especially for those at risk; safer sex education; a TB test within the first three months of membership and again annually for every member; substance abuse screening and MISA programs at each location; tardive dyskinesia screening (see Chapter Two); dental, vision, and hearing screening; stress management groups; a weight control program and nutrition education; and a smoking cessation program.

Overall, we estimate that we are at about 60 percent of where we would like to be in meeting our physical health goal. Additionally, we are not optimistic about smoking cessation and weight control, based on our experience in these areas. Nicotine addiction is particularly intractable, although all our day facilities are smoke free. We have had a "health month" that emphasized physical exams, a smoking cessation day, walking and other forms of exercise, meal planning for good health, and extensive blood work (including HIV testing for those willing to be tested). We are seriously concerned about HIV/AIDS because psychiatric patients are a major risk group. Undoubtedly this will be a focus of future program efforts. One concern rests with members' reactions to the news that they are HIV positive. Some deny being positive, even after several tests, and others become angry and resume sexual activity; counseling assumes great importance.

Value of Goals

Having clear goals offers many advantages in organizing a program. Our six goals provide a focus for staff and member goal setting and meaningful participation. They are the touchstones of our comprehensive approach, and to top it off, they make good sense from a practical point of view. When we evaluate the effect of the total program, we examine how well individual members have done in whatever goals they have chosen to work on, and we look at how well the agency as a whole is performing in delivering the goal-related services it wants to deliver.

References

Bond, G. R., and Dincin, J. "Accelerating Entry into Transitional Employment in a Psychosocial Rehabilitation Agency." *Rehabilitation Psychology*, 1986, *31*, 143–155.

Dincin, J. "Housing: A Crucial Dimension." *National Rehabilitation Association: 1988 Switzer Monograph.* Washington, D.C.: U.S. Government Printing Office, 1988.

Stein, L. I., and Test, M. A. (eds.). *The Training in Community Living Model: A Decade of Experience.* New Directions for Mental Health Services, no. 26. San Francisco: Jossey-Bass, 1985.

Witheridge, T. F., and Dincin, J. "The Assertive Community Treatment Worker: An Emerging Role and Its Implications for Professional Training." *Hospital and Community Psychiatry,* 1985, *40* (6), 620–624.

JERRY DINCIN is executive director of Thresholds.

Special groups of persons with mental illness require
individually tailored programs.

Special Programs for Special Groups

Jerry Dincin, Mary Ann Zeitz, Diane Farrell,
Linda Harrington, Walter Green, Debbie Pavick,
Camille Rucks, Peter Illing

The lobby of Thresholds North bursts with activity as the doors officially open at 8:30 A.M. The action comes from more than the influx of members and staff into our day programming. A group of mothers with their young children fill the first floor with youthful voices and energy. They are part of the Thresholds Mothers Project, one of several specialized programs that have grown explosively during the last fifteen years in response to the special needs of particular groups. When needed, psychiatric rehabilitation at Thresholds has transformed itself from the usual clubhouse model as programming has been adapted for these special groups in many different ways over the years. What has resulted is a plethora of innovative and exciting programs, including several one-of-a-kind programs.

The program for the hearing impaired developed because no one was serving the deaf community. The Mothers Project developed when it became clear that a member was neglecting her two-year-old. The Young Adult Program developed because several eighteen-year-olds were unsuccessful in the adult program. The Thresholds Bridge Program for the Homeless project developed because many in the burgeoning population of homeless have a history of mental illness. The program for members with both a mental illness and a substance abuse problem developed because of the tremendous influx of these dually diagnosed people. The Older Adult Program is a response to those with psychiatric illness who also have significant issues associated with aging. Some programs were built on the germs of ideas sprouted elsewhere (the Bridge programs and the Mothers Project). Other were born of a staff member's personal commitment (the Program for Deaf and Mentally Ill Persons) (Kozlowski-

Graham, 1991). Yet others grew from a perceived need in the whole field of psychiatric rehabilitation (the homeless program) or in Thresholds services particularly (the program for mentally ill substance abusers). In this chapter, the staff members who direct these special or niche programs describe each of them.

While these programs account for a large portion of Thresholds' growth over the past fifteen years, they also tend to be more expensive to operate than typical psychiatric rehabilitation day programs because they require a greater number of staff and also staff with unique skills. However, Thresholds was able to spur their growth by being open to new ideas, being willing to start small, utilizing unusual funding sources, searching out invested program leaders who were willing to step up to take responsibility, and of course, having some good luck.

At this moment, Thresholds is considering four other groups of clients for whom services are lacking in Illinois: the mentally ill and mentally retarded; the mentally ill and physically disabled; the mentally ill populations in county jails or in forensic institutions for the mentally ill, and severely emotionally disturbed children under sixteen years of age. Time, funding opportunities, staff commitment, and board decisions will determine what will happen in these areas.

Mothers Project

Mary Ann Zeitz

The Mothers Project was begun in 1976 as a research and demonstration program, funded by the National Institute of Mental Health, for mothers with mental illness and their children between the ages of two months and five years. Funds from many private foundations, particularly the Crown Foundation and the Fred Woods Memorial, along with monies from Thresholds itself, kept the program functioning for ten years, at which time further government funds became available.

The underlying philosophy of the Mothers Project is that before a mother is able to meet the needs of her growing child, her own needs must be met. The women in this project often feel depleted by their mental illness and need to experience empathy and caring from staff before they can adequately respond to their children. The project's special goals (in addition to the six Thresholds goals) are to provide crisis intervention, to teach better parenting skills, to form a peer group from these socially isolated women, and to provide emotional support in the form of caring and consistent limit setting. Because the children in this program are vulnerable to cognitive and psychiatric disorders, we provide primary intervention services through a sophisticated nursery that makes careful diagnostic and developmental assessments and then offers remediation and treatment.

Program staff began their work with mothers who were wards of the Illinois Department of Children and Family Services (DCFS) because it had become apparent that intervention services were vital for these women, who were themselves neglected or abused as children. These mothers are between the ages of eighteen and twenty-one, are pregnant or parenting, have mental illness, and exhibit impaired functioning. The program also works with families who have lost custody of their children solely owing to an episode of mental illness, instances that have quickly made it clear that child welfare officials have not understood the impact of mental illness on parenting. Staff advocate for these families in a "best interest of the child" context that holds that the needs of the child must be primary but that the child is usually best cared for within the family of origin if possible.

Another program in the Mothers Project funded by the DCFS provides therapeutic day care services for fifteen young children. The admission criteria are that the mother have serious mental illness and that the referring source indicate that the child and/or the child's development is at risk because of the mother's psychopathology. This program addresses its services to older, more chronically ill women who are trying their best to parent and provide for their children, despite their own continuing symptoms.

The entire Mothers Project is unique because of the comprehensive services it offers that are especially important to women with young children. The mothers participate in the five-day-a-week therapeutic nursery according to their individual service plans and are then able to pursue their personal rehabilitation program at the same site. We have found through the years that this psychiatric rehabilitation program offers women with young children a special path to functioning not available elsewhere. A vocational component is especially tailored for each mother, so that she can move at her own pace, beginning with a situational assessment on-site and continuing with work adjustment and job development services that are sensitive to her role as a mother. These mothers, in particular, make use of the Thresholds education program, working toward GEDs and learning basic literacy skills, which are increasingly important for the mothers not only as they learn about independent living but also as they assist their own children with learning fundamentals. The social program, including participation in the Child Development Group, Mothers Therapy Group, and the Stress Management and the Health Issues Groups, offers opportunities to enhance self-esteem and has positive effects on the mother-child relationship.

In its case management aspect, the program can be representative payee in order to manage mothers' funds and to teach much-needed budgeting skills. Of course, each mother is helped to obtain all appropriate state and federal funding to which she and her child are entitled. All medical services necessary to mother and child are arranged by the program, including prenatal through postnatal services and contraceptive information and materials. Psychiatric services are provided by the agency's consulting psychiatrists and medication compliance is stressed. Besides mental illness, some women in the Mothers Project are also confronting substance abuse. The program offers on-site education and support groups several times per week on these issues. In addition, on-site testing equipment is available to detect alcohol, cocaine and derivatives, marijuana, and PCP use.

The program also provides activities available to "normal" families. Staff often become the extended family for these mothers and children as they learn to celebrate holidays together and go on field trips that offer nuturance for both mother and child as well as a normalizing activity. The comprehensiveness of this treatment program is truly unique, involving treatment of the mother, of the child, and of the mother-child relationship at the same time and in the same place. We emphasize that treatment of the mother is aimed at increasing her ability to effectively parent her child. Even the material used in the academic program has childrearing as its subject. The parent remains on-site at all times and is immediately accessible to her child.

From the merest speck of an idea, born out of the perceived hardship of two members, this program has developed into a strong, comprehensive, and much-needed service. Much more needs to be done throughout the United States for mentally ill mothers and their children, and there is a major opportunity for future expansion in this area at all psychiatric rehabilitation agencies that are capable of providing the best blend of services and commitment.

Research on the Mothers Project. In the original Mothers Project funded by a research and demonstration grant, women were randomly assigned to the agency component with its therapeutic nursery and psychosocial approach, a home-visiting outreach program, and a control group. Results indicated that both the agency-based and outreach components were more effective than the control services (Stott and others, 1984). These two elements were later combined into the two basic services of clubhouse programs and assertive outreach psychosocial rehabilitation skills training and support. Of the forty mothers served in 1994, only four (10 percent) had psychiatric hospitalizations during that year. Client satisfaction data collected in fiscal year 1994 indicated overall high levels of member approval of the program (Cook, Urwin, and Osborne, 1994). All the women said they would recommend the program to a woman "in need of similar help," and all also indicated that they would turn to the program if they were to "seek help again" in the future. Follow-up data collected six months after program exit (Cook and Razzano, 1995) found that 90 percent of the women had avoided psychiatric hospitalization since leaving the Mothers Project and three-quarters (76 percent) were living in commercially available housing at that time. One-third had been employed during the follow-up period. Overall, the Mothers Project helps women avoid psychiatric hospitalization, live independently, and pursue life goals for themselves, their children, and their families.

In fiscal year 1994, the Mothers Project served 106 mothers, children, and fathers with sixteen staff and a budget of $620,000.

Young Adult Program

Diane Farrell

In 1974, Thresholds recognized that the needs of older adolescents with psychiatric problems were not being met adequately in programs originally designed for adults. In response, Thresholds established the Young Adult Program (YAP), predicated on the thesis that older adolescents (sixteen to twenty-one years old) need to be involved in comprehensive age-appropriate programming designed for them and only for them.

The Young Adult Program is essentially a microcosm of the traditional Thresholds model, adhering to all the key elements of psychiatric rehabilitation but modified to be more effective for adolescents.

Funding for the YAP is rather different than for the rest of the agency. A per diem rate is established by a state agency for both the YAP day program and the YAP residential program, and these fees are typically paid by several boards of education, the DCFS, and the Illinois Department of Mental Health (DMH) and occasionally by out-of-state referrals, insurance, and managed care companies.

Originally, the YAP coexisted in the same physical facility as the Adult Program at Thresholds North. Because this was an uneasy coexistence for all, the board of directors accepted the need for a free-standing physical plant that would be more appropriate and effective for adolescent programs and undertook a $2 million capital campaign to finance that project. In 1990, the YAP moved triumphantly, during a blizzard, into its own location. The new facility incorporates the clubhouse model of physical space: a living room, kitchen, dining room, crew areas, and so on, but also has classrooms, a computer lab, a large gymnasium, an area devoted to group rooms, and several areas devoted to recreational use. The YAP atmosphere differs from that of other programs. Upon entering the building, you will find the living room empty but the recreational areas jammed, active, and noisy.

The YAP is a modification of the usual psychiatric rehabilitation model, since it has a much stronger psychotherapeutic component. Case workers do therapy in addition to providing the traditional case management services. This is necessary and critical if older adolescents are to develop effective coping skills and avoid chronicity. The YAP is a viable alternative to hospitalization, which is too often the traditional first step of psychiatric treatment for the troubled adolescent. Instead, every possible option should be explored to provide effective and cost-conscious treatment that will lead an adolescent along the path toward health with as little hospitalization as possible. The YAP addresses the key developmental tasks of adolescence for older adolescents with mental illness and/or severe behavioral disorders; provides structure in all program components; carefully balances limit setting and nurturing (the key to working effectively with adolescents); and emphasizes group, individual, and family therapy.

The YAP operates a licensed, accredited high school with a six-to-one student/teacher ratio. All teachers are trained in special education and can also provide for the needs of those with learning disabilities. Credits earned in the YAP school may be applied to Thresholds graduation requirements or transferred to the adolescent's home school. Either way, the adolescent is able to earn a high school diploma. Completion of a high school diploma, development of skills and competencies, and mastery are primary concerns of both the adolescents and the YAP educational staff. Teachers are fully integrated into the milieu and, to the greatest extent possible, function within the typical psychiatric rehabilitation model for generalist staff.

The Thresholds social program is the core of the YAP, providing an opportunity for all members to establish a sense of belonging, a sense of purpose, and a feeling of hope and to learn the tools to promote personal growth and change. Indeed, the YAP is founded on the belief that the primary agent of change for adolescents is the group. Group process remains a central ingredient of all aspects of the program planning, and many different groups are run during the three afternoons a week devoted to group activities.

It is always difficult to describe the social programs within psychiatric rehabilitation programs and the social power of groups. Additional components of our social program that enrich and enhance the group experience are camping trips, field trips, the annual school graduation ceremony, parties and dances, an annual twenty-four-hour fundraiser, and a prom.

Although we believe in the importance of group process for troubled adolescents, and always strive to nurture this process, we also believe strongly in the value of our style of individual therapy for these young people. All members have the opportunity to participate in individual therapy within the agency. In addition, family contact is initiated and maintained for each YAP member, and family counseling is conducted as desired and necessary.

The vocational component essentially follows the same guidelines in the YAP as it does in other Thresholds programs. The main difference is added structure: we utilize a behavioral management "levels system" within our vocational crews and our residential program. Job placement programs are similarly structured.

The YAP currently operates four group homes, with a fifth to open soon. Each home operates on an objective behavioral system, so as to facilitate development of internal controls. The structure provided allows members to guide and perceive their growth through a system encompassing responsibilities, mandatory behaviors, privileges, natural cause-and-effect consequences, positive expectations, and peer support. The graduated levels system increases responsibility and privileges through various successes in skill development. Group process is an integral feature of this approach.

When we have visitors to the YAP, the tour is always conducted by a staff person and a member because we believe that members' words best convey the true sense of what Thresholds is all about. For example, listen to these comments from several different youngsters: "Thresholds tries to teach us that we are worthy of love and that we can be whatever we want to be"; "Staff are gentle and caring and show you that love and trust are just there for the asking"; "Thresholds to me is people—people who want nothing more from me than to see me grow and be happy"; "At Thresholds if you give of yourself, it will give to you"; "The Young Adult Program is not only a special place . . . it is a place to feel special."

Research on the Young Adult Program. Research on the young adult program suggests that it maintains a low rate of hospitalization among members at the same time that it helps youths attain other life goals. This was shown in an analysis of employment and hospitalization rates in the YAP in the years before and after implementing a model vocational program (Cook and others, in press). The proportion employed rose steadily, from 44 percent of all young adults in the year before program implementation to 56 percent at the end of the first year of the program and 58 percent at the end of the second year. During that same time, the proportion hospitalized remained stable: 23 percent the year prior to the program and 17 percent and 21 percent at the end of the first and second years of the program respectively. This suggests that the YAP helps older adolescents avoid relapses into their psychiatric disability at the same time that it assists them in attaining adult life goals.

The Young Adult Program has been the focus of much research since its inception (see Chapter Six), including longitudinal studies of employment (Cook, Solomon, and Mock, 1989), studies of effects of therapeutic camping (Farrell, 1982), studies of results of a visiting chefs program (Roussel and Cook, 1987), and studies of improvement in mathematics and reading scores following classroom instruction (Willerman, Wessell, and Cook, 1986).

In fiscal year 1994, the Thresholds Young Adult Program served about ninety-eight members with thirty-four full-time staff, and a yearly operating budget of $1,850,000. About sixty members are served at any one time.

Program for Deaf and Mentally Ill Persons

Linda Harrington

In Illinois, advocates for the deaf community had begun organizing as early as 1979 on behalf of deaf persons with mental illness who were institutionalized for long periods of time in state hospitals without adequate access to signed communication or treatment. These advocates, from a variety of agencies and professions, with the added pressure of a possible American Civil Liberties Union lawsuit, eventually secured a commitment from the DMH to develop a single inpatient psychiatric unit for deaf persons and to provide funding for comprehensive community treatment. Thresholds was the first agency the DMH approached in search of services and programming, and Thresholds has led the field in the development of a continuum of care for deaf adults with severe and persistent mental illness.

An excellent model of a continuum of care exists between the state hospital inpatient unit and Thresholds outpatient services. In many ways, it has developed as an ideal, relatively seamless model, in which Thresholds staff are consulted as inpatients improve and before they are considered for discharge. These consultations involve both inpatient treatment direction and outpatient plans and allow for intelligent integrated decision making with mutual respect on both sides. In a similar way, there is no hassle when Thresholds needs to hospitalize one of its residents. This good working relationship exists with state hospitals at most Thresholds programs, but it is within the deaf program that the often-discussed but seldom-manifested continuum of care works best.

The deaf program offers a wide array of services including twenty-four-hour supervised group homes, home visiting, and job support. The program currently consists of three residences, two assertive community treatment teams, and a vocational team. All these teams offer different services to the membership. The three residences all use the group home model. Each, however, has adapted the model to meet residents' special needs. The most staff-intensive residence, Kiley House, can work with persons with the triple diagnosis of mental illness, deafness, and developmental disability. These members need much structure and supervision in order to perform their daily living tasks adequately. The house is staffed accordingly. California House, a step toward greater independence, has shift staff awake twenty-four hours but offers fewer hours of day programming in the residence. Residents have more free time and interact more independently in the community. The program direction in these two residences is geared toward improving communication skills, activities of daily living (money management, travel, cooking), and substance abuse education. Most of the activities found in the usual Thresholds day program are replicated but with a special relevance for the deaf. For instance, frustration tolerance is low for many of the members in these two residences, and that fact needs to be addressed consistently. Washtenaw House is the third phase of independence for deaf members. The live-in manager is a sleep-over and an evening activity worker. Residents are expected to have a job, attend school or other programs outside the house during the day, and return in the evening for a communal meal. Members who demonstrate the living skills necessary to live independently in the community are placed in apartments not affiliated with Thresholds and receive regular visits from an assertive community treatment team and the full range of long-term Bridge-type case management services as needed.

A member living in any type of housing situation is eligible to receive services from the vocational team if he or she chooses. These services include, but are not limited to, group and individual job placement, help with placement in competitive jobs in the community, in-house job support groups, referral to community colleges, and sheltered workshop employment. An important goal of the vocational team is to train members to work as staff within the deaf program itself. It is our belief that we demonstrate to employers the value of the work of our members when we want to hire them ourselves!

For decades, deaf mentally ill persons were considered to be uneducable or untreatable. We have demonstrated this perception to be erroneous. Persons who spent most of their adult lives in institutions are now living in the community. Persons who once called the state hospital home now reserve that title for their own apartment or their room in our residence. Persons who once depended upon disability payments to support themselves are now working independently and paying taxes. The Thresholds Program for Deaf and Mentally Ill Persons has demonstrated that psychiatric rehabilitation works. In fact, the program has been able to accept occasional referrals from public agencies in states that do not have a similar program and occasionally from private families who will pay for comprehensive, well-organized, and effective services for this specialized group.

Research on the deaf program. Research on the Program for Deaf and Mentally Ill Persons indicates that it helps members avoid psychiatric hospitalization while improving their independent living and employment outcomes and lowering their levels of psychiatric symptoms. Analysis of outcomes among the program's first sixty clients served between May 1984 and August 1989 (Cook, Kozlowski-Graham, and Razzano, 1993) found improvement in several outcome areas. Over half had worked for pay at some time during their participation (10 percent were employed at intake), 45 percent of all members lived in a commercially available community residence during the program (only 20 percent had done so at intake), and 43 percent remained free of further psychiatric hospitalizations after entering the program (as a group, they averaged 5.8 admissions at intake).

In addition, significant improvements were noted in a group of twenty-five deaf clients followed up after one year of service delivery (Kozlowski-Graham, Cook, and Razzano, 1995). These members had significantly lower levels of psychiatric symptoms than at intake; they also were less functionally impaired after one year in the program. Their independent living skills and social participation rates increased significantly over their intake levels. Finally, these members reported significantly lower feelings of stigma about their deafness and their psychiatric disability as compared to their feelings at intake. Although the threat of regression to the mean suggests caution in interpreting these results, deaf program members do appear to show positive changes, and sizable proportions achieve outcomes that enhance their community living.

In fiscal year 1994, this program served eighty-three people, using twenty-five staff, and a budget of $1,474,000.

Short-Term Program for Homeless Mentally Ill Persons: Mobile Assessment Unit

Walter Green

The Thresholds Mobile Assessment Unit (MAU) was the first program of its kind in Chicago (and one of the few in the nation) specifically designed to address the needs of mentally ill homeless people while they are still on the streets. The essential tasks performed by MAU staff are short-term outreach, engagement, crisis intervention, assessment, referral, and linkage. Services are time limited: the goal is to provide the supports necessary to enable mentally ill homeless people to make a quick and smooth transition from the streets to housing and then to other mental health and supportive services, including Thresholds' long-term homeless team.

MAU staff, consisting of six outreach workers, a secretary/dispatcher, and the program director, work with homeless persons anywhere in Chicago. The outreach workers include two licensed clinical social workers/qualified examiners—who, under Illinois law, can execute a certificate for involuntary hospitalization—one M.S.W., and three bachelor's-level staff, all of whom can execute a petition for involuntary hospitalization.

The program operates Monday through Friday, from 8:00 A.M. to 4:00 P.M. After a brief morning meeting to plan the day, the staff "hit the streets." Staff work in three teams of two, but there is no fixed composition to the dyads other than that the two L.C.S.W.'s generally do not ride together. Working in dyads is a necessity because the teams operate in an unstructured environment with seriously mentally ill people whom they do not know, and staff safety must be a serious consideration. Significantly, however, no MAU staff person has ever been injured on the job.

Once in the field, the teams make contact with clients through two methods. A "cold call" is a direct approach to a person on the street or in an abandoned building, an underground haunt, or one of Chicago's many parks. In warm weather, a dyad is often assigned to do outreach via bicycle in the parks, where vehicles are prohibited. The other method of intake is a referral from a shelter provider or other agency. Referrals are phoned into the Mobile Assessment Unit office crisis line, where the dispatcher takes the basic information and contacts the staff via two-way radio. As the teams are already in the field, response time can be very rapid.

Whether first contact with a person is made via outreach or referral, an initial mental health assessment is conducted and a service plan is developed for that person. Because many variables must be considered in each assessment—such as current level of functioning, past mental health, and resources in the area, to name but a few—each plan is custom made. Here, too, the value of working in dyads is apparent, since each initial assessment invariably requires numerous phone calls to identify and coordinate services.

The possible outcomes of the initial assessment also cover a broad spectrum. Hospitalization is initiated about 25 percent of the time; 80 percent of these hospitalizations are voluntary admissions, and the remainder are accomplished through certificate and/or petition. MAU staff then work with the member and the hospital staff to establish an appropriate discharge plan, including linkage to mental health services, entitlements, and housing. Although the need for housing is obvious, MAU staff often encounter people who have been discharged from a state or community hospital directly to the streets.

Hospitalization is in many ways an ideal outcome for this population and would be more often initiated but for the great difficulty of getting people without funding into a hospital. In addition to the advantage of providing immediate psychiatric stabilization, hospitalization also gives MAU staff the luxury of knowing where a member is for a fixed period of time, making it much easier to arrange appointments and coordinate resources.

Representing the majority of the MAU's work are those initial assessments where the member refuses services, often as a result of paranoia. Indeed, some first contacts yield no more than observations of people who refuse to speak to the team. It is important to note that the refusal of services is almost always a symptom of illness and does not constitute "choosing" to live on the streets. For these members, MAU staff have developed some simple engagement techniques that yield remarkable results.

The key to successful engagement with the homeless mentally ill who present with initial resistance has proven to be staff capacity to provide immediate and concrete services that address basic needs. Those people who know the Thresholds name are wary of any mention of mental health services but will often accept food, clothing, a shower, or a night in a single room occupancy hotel. Mobile Assessment Unit staff have learned to be extremely flexible in addressing a person's expressed needs.

An essential element in successful outreach and engagement with the homeless mentally ill is finding out what the person values and then making it a top priority to meet that need. Of equal importance is how the need is met—whenever possible it is done with no strings attached. An attitude of unconditional positive regard is absolutely as critical with people on the streets as it is in any other rehabilitative relationship—perhaps more so. Many homeless mentally ill individuals relate stories of abuse and neglect, of the violation of their rights, of the failure of mental health professionals to treat them with respect. Mobile Assessment Unit staff often witness this abuse firsthand, directed at people who may be dirty or identified as "treatment resistant," a label often used by providers as justification for refusing to offer services. Thus, after beginning to gain the person's trust, an essential element of a MAU worker's job is to advocate for that person's right to treatment. Anyone who attempts to secure services for a homeless mentally ill person should expect one or more hostile encounters with other service providers. As one administrator informed MAU's program director, "The problem with your clients is that they're usually very dirty and very crazy, and my staff don't like working with them." Regrettably, this attitude is as much the norm as not.

In spite of these obstacles, MAU staff experience clearly demonstrates that even the most difficult among the homeless mentally ill, for example, persons who have been homeless and unmedicated for as long as ten years, will accept services and treatment if staff are willing to be creative, flexible, and persistent in meeting that person's needs.

Research on the Mobile Assessment Unit. Research findings suggest that the MAU program deflects a large majority of its clients from hospital admission. Data on 1,430 members served during a two-year period beginning in July 1990 (Slagg and others, 1994) indicate that only 21 percent were hospitalized, half of them (10 percent) voluntarily. An additional study examined the effects of using mental health consumers as MAU staff (Lyons and others, in press). This research revealed very few differences between consumer and nonconsumer staff in the nature and outcomes of services delivered or in clients, suggesting that consumers were indistinguishable in their effects on the service delivery model. One interesting difference was that consumer dyads (those with one or both consumer members) engaged in significantly more street outreach than did nonconsumer dyads. It may be that consumer staff are more motivated to engage in assertive outreach, spending less time in the office and more out on the streets. Overall, the research suggests that consumers can perform as well as nonconsumers in delivering mobile crisis assessment services.

In fiscal year 1994, the Mobile Assessment Unit provided services to 409 people with eight full-time staff and a budget of $396,000.

Long-Term Bridge Program for the Homeless Mentally Ill: Assertive Community Treatment

Debbie Pavick

In the mid to late 1980s, the plight of the homeless became increasingly obvious as more and more people were observed sleeping on the streets, going through garbage dumpsters, and carrying their bags of belongings about with them. Among these homeless individuals, many exhibited behaviors that were bizarre or socially inappropriate and usually an indication of a mental illness. Though there has always been controversy over the total number of homeless persons, it is generally accepted that persons with severe and persistent mental illness make up approximately one-third of the homeless population (Task Force on Homelessness and Severe Mental Illness, 1992). The high visibility of homeless mentally ill in our society pointed to gaps in the current system of delivery of mental health care and drew the attention of policy makers. Funding became available for development of programs specific to this population.

In 1987, Thresholds Bridge North program was awarded special funding from the City of Chicago and the DMH to set up a six-person team of outreach workers to provide long-term assertive community treatment (ACT) for sixty homeless mentally ill persons. Thresholds had not yet had a program dedicated exclusively to serving the needs of the homeless, but we believed that the key features of the Thresholds Bridge model (see Chapter Four) were transferable to this population. The Bridge North program's original mission had been to serve the highest users of psychiatric hospitals and prevent their rehospitalization, and it was a natural extension of that mission to include persons who were both homeless and mentally ill.

We realized that engagement, though always a process, would take on new meaning, as this was a significantly more disenfranchised population than even the most frequently hospitalized individuals in our existing membership. Few homeless persons had any current connections to family, medical, or psychiatric care. They had no reason to believe that we would offer anything different than previous helpers in a system that perpetually failed them.

After the engagement process between a homeless mentally ill person and Thresholds Bridge North was well underway, the intake complete, housing found, and weekly home visits scheduled, the team's focus remained task oriented. Staff found that this population had health problems directly related to or exacerbated by life on the streets and that much time was spent accompanying members to medical appointments. Most members, due largely to problems with substance abuse, needed Thresholds to act as representative payee for their Social Security benefits to ensure that their rent was paid and that there was food money for the entire month. Substance use also decreased when members were not given cash but instead were accompanied by a staff person when purchasing clothing or groceries. Our accepting ultimate responsibility was not only a key for linking program members to services but also helpful in cultivating a wide spectrum of housing. Landlords, room-and-board houses, and single room occupancy hotel managers were more open to housing our members sight unseen because of our willingness to provide ongoing home visits and accept responsibility when problems arose. Once program members were housed, more time was spent teaching them and assisting them with basic activities of daily living. Whereas in other programs, a staff person might make a quick check of a member's room and engage him or her in conversation over a cup of coffee, these members needed active staff assistance with medication monitoring, basic personal hygiene, laundry, and room cleaning.

Serving the needs of these members was made easier by the addition of a psychiatric consultant and a general practitioner to our treatment team. Both professionals are committed to serving our members and do not shy away from them even when they come directly from the streets or a shelter. The psychiatrist is available to see new members weekly and will make home visits if requested by the program. The general practitioner sees everyone after intake and annually for a complete physical examination. For those members whose Medicaid application is in process, he has agreed to accept delayed payment for services rendered.

The essential ingredient of our success in preventing Thresholds Bridge North members from returning to homelessness is the accessibility of our services via one door. That is to say, we are the conduit through which they obtain comprehensive care. A major role of the program outreach worker is to directly provide or broker services in a system where supports and resources are fragmented and difficult of access. The current delivery system in most places requires the homeless mentally ill to link with a multitude of service providers for their physical and emotional well-being. Funding, housing, and psychiatric and medical care all exist as separate entities, each with various rules and requests, a situation that confounds even the highest-functioning homeless person. The mentally ill person whose thinking is disorganized and who is paranoid is unable to negotiate the many bureaucracies where resources exist. Basic survival, looking for food and a safe place to sleep, takes precedence over trying to access entitlement benefits. Even if these people make it through the door of an agency, withstand the long wait, and finally get seen, they may be turned away for not having a state ID or a birth certificate, documents that can only be attained by negotiating with yet other bureaucracies.

The techniques for accomplishing our mission call for nothing fancy, just a willingness to engage in a nitty-gritty, time-consuming, and labor-intensive approach. A team sensitive to the varied characteristics and long-term course of homeless persons with severe mental illness and able to provide in vivo support and integrate a wide array of services can prevent homelessness and hopelessness and improve the quality of life over the long term for the homeless mentally ill. We must be prepared to stay with them, offering service, if need be, for their entire lives.

Research on Thresholds Bridge North for the Homeless. At the Thresholds Bridge North for the Homeless project, research conducted for the Illinois Department of Mental Health and Developmental Disabilities (DMHDD) (Korr and Joseph, 1994) compared homeless DMHDD inpatients randomly assigned to Bridge versus "treatment as usual." After six months of services, 75 percent of the Bridge group were stably housed compared to only 34 percent of the controls, a statistically significant difference. After one year of services, the proportion of Bridge members housed remained high at 69 percent, while many of the control group could not even be located to assess their housing status. A comparison of state rehospitalization statistics between all Bridge clients and those in the control group indicated that Bridge clients experienced a 60 percent reduction in average number of bed-days, from sixty-two days per client in the year prior to twenty-five days per client in the year after. Conversely, the control group showed a much smaller reduction of only 26 percent, from seventy-nine days per client in the year prior to fifty-eight days per client in the year after. Thus, Bridge services to homeless members help them find and retain community housing at the same time as they reduce use of psychiatric inpatient services.

This long-term Bridge program for the homeless mentally ill served sixty-one people with fifteen full-time staff and a budget of $507,000 in fiscal year 1994.

Program for Mentally Ill Substance Abusers

Camille Rucks

It had become apparent over a ten-year period that substance abuse among Thresholds members was becoming an epidemic, and we were ill prepared to cope with the problems of mentally ill substance abuser (MISA) members. In our state, substance abuse clinics do not want to work with persons with severe mental illness, and mental health agencies have been both reluctant and naïve in regard to substance abuse treatment.

The Thresholds response was to form an agency task force that studied the issue for a year. The group read articles, visited exemplary programs, and attended professional meetings and conferences in order to formulate a philosophy and program. In this program's philosophy, abstinence is not a requirement for the program, and members' relapse experiences are seen as learning opportunities rather than reasons for negative consequences.

Thresholds has always been an agency that focuses on members' individual needs. Staff look at members' unique strengths and limitations in combination with their resources, environments, and cultural identities when formulating treatment plans. This same procedure was determined to be important with our MISA members as well. One-on-one work with members who have addiction or substance abuse problems is crucial.

The MISA program does not assume that members will follow a linear pathway to recovery but rather that recovery is typically a nonlinear process, with the insight and ability to remain drug and alcohol free developing over time. Staff, we decided, would need to be flexible in allowing members to take advantage of vocational, educational, social, and residential opportunities during this process. Of course, all MISA members would be scheduled into as much of the MISA programming as they could effectively use, and many, we expected, would probably need to have drug and alcohol testing built into their treatment plan at some point. As a result of this study group's work, important additions were made to the basic Thresholds program so that the agency could serve MISA members. These additions include the following:

Day program enhancements. The CAGE (Cut, Annoyed, Guilty, & Eye-Opener) questionnaire is administered to all Thresholds members at the point of intake. Additionally, each member is administered a screening tool (the MISA Checklist) designed to detect addiction or abuse problems. Those members who display the traits of abuse or addiction are referred to specialized groups and programs that creatively address their needs.

Group program components. The MISA program consists of day program groups and linkage to outside twelve-step recovery and support groups. Some of the groups are didactic, with drug and alcohol education as their main goal. Others are supportive and therapeutic. Still others are available to the relatives of MISA members, to help them in their stressful roles of coping with a dually diagnosed friend or relative. The titles of the day program groups are Substance Abuse Education Group, Substance Abuse Treatment Group, STEMSS (Support Together for Emotional and Mental Sobriety and Serenity) Group, Relapse Prevention Group, and Parent/Family Support and Education Group.

Testing for drug use. Despite our best efforts, we know that members who have an addiction or abuse problem also have a high rate of relapse and that members will continue to deny the problem as part and parcel of the disease known as addiction. Drug testing in the agency can help somewhat in preventing and detecting relapse and denial. Drug-testing kits and Breathalyzers are available at each Thresholds branch and are voluntary. Local hospitals are the screening sites for more complex testing.

Residential program. Thresholds existing residential programs were not adequate to meet the needs of most members with an abuse or addiction problem. The MISA task force investigated residential programs for people who have a chemical dependency (CD) and combined the ideology and methods used in both CD residential programming and traditional Thresholds group homes to create the MISA group home.

Thresholds operates three MISA group homes for eight members each. All have a dual diagnosis and have failed in their rehabilitation attempts due to use of alcohol and/or street drugs. The expected length of stay in the group home is about one year. Various groups, such as the Substance Abuse Education, Treatment Group, Relapse Prevention Group, and STEMSS Group, are provided in the group home. Additional groups focus on basic rehabilitation issues such as independent living skills, stress management, and medication compliance. Again, while some of the groups are didactic, others help members recognize that it is possible to have fun in a sober state. Individual treatment is also an integral component of the MISA group home. Each member is assigned a staff worker upon entry, meeting at least weekly with the worker to discuss issues of recovery and rehabilitation. The treatment team works with the member to design an individualized treatment program based on changes the member needs to make for a drug- and alcohol-free life-style and other personal long-term goals.

Members in this program also operate under a levels system in the group home. Compliance with the treatment plan earns the member time to self-structure and added responsibilities and privileges. When a member enters the MISA group home, he or she is under twenty-four-hour staff supervision for the first thirty days. After that time, the member can begin to move up the level system.

The MISA residential program is designed to be comprehensive enough so that the residents need not join the day program at a Thresholds branch in order to achieve success in any of the six goal areas. MISA members use the group home as their personal day program. However, members may make use of the other Thresholds residences or day programs after their tenure in the MISA group home.

Staff training. The MISA task force decided that rather than recruiting staff from outside addiction programs to operate the MISA program, it would be more efficient and effective to train existing staff in the areas of addiction and dual diagnosis.

There is no research yet on this new program. The capacity of the three MISA group homes is twenty-four persons, with a staff of sixteen and a budget of $775,000.

Older Adult Program

Peter Illing

Once the older psychiatric patients at Thresholds were identified as a group in need of specialized services, we searched for a model of such services. Mike Bernstein's three-part system at Gulf Coast Jewish Family Service was chosen after we made a productive and informative visit there. Over the long term, we envision replicating all three parts of the system: day services within a partial hospitalization program (PHP), a residential component in the form of an enlarged group home, and a consultation service to nursing homes. At the moment, we have only the PHP, started in late 1994, in place.

Some members of the Older Adult Program have had severe mental ill-ness since their teens or twenties. Others have had moderate mental illness but have continued to live with their families through their life cycles. These peo-ple had never had the opportunity to learn to live with some self-reliance, to succeed or fail in normal tasks of adulthood, and now crises were occurring or looming as their immediate family members died and support dwindled. Another group has had mild or moderate mental illness later in the life cycle. As the people in this group aged and experienced loss of functioning, physi-cal decline, and new developmental demands, the stress became sufficient to trigger mental illness.

On the surface, the needs of the elderly mentally ill appeared the same as those of their younger peers. Improved psychiatric stability, a meaningful pro-ductive role, social support and stimulation, supportive housing, attention to physical health concerns and avoidance of substance abuse were seen as legit-imate goals. However, these goals have different meanings and priorities for the older adult, who operates out of a more reflective viewpoint and tends to be more cautious and self-doubting. In addition, these older members are more accepting of their limitations and illnesses.

One foundation and one individual donor each provided a modest three-year grant as seed money for the Older Adult Program at Thresholds. In June 1994, a program director was hired, and the program opened in October 1994. The current program consists of five days per week of intensive partial hospi-talization day treatment. The minimum age of participants has been set at fifty-five. The program functions as an alternative for individuals who were already members at Thresholds but who were experiencing special problems due to age, developmental difficulties, or goal attainment. Other members are referred from intermediate care facilities and nursing homes. The six Thresholds goals have been adapted to the needs of this special group: the program is intended to help members find meaning, satisfaction, and happiness in their lives; prevent psy-chiatric hospitalization; ameliorate symptoms of mental illness; continue life skills development; encourage older adult developmental tasks; develop each individual's capacity for independence and interdependence; and increase well-being through personalized physical, mental, social, and spiritual activity.

The day-to-day functioning of the program is heavily influenced by the dominating effects of physical illness, psychiatric disability, and lack of stamina in these older members' lives. Every member uses medication both for a phys-ical illness and a psychiatric condition. The majority have difficulty with atten-tion and alertness due to advanced age. This has several program implications. Members must frequently be excused from day program attendance to attend medical appointments. Virtually every case management session devotes some time to reviewing health and to medical follow-up. The origin and the needed treatment of symptoms are frequently clouded with uncertainty, and as one would expect, management of psychotropic medication is more complicated than in a younger population.

So far the Older Adult Program has served eighteen people with four staff.

References

Cook, J. A., Kozlowski-Graham, K., and Razzano, L. "Psychosocial Rehabilitation of Deaf Persons with Severe Mental Illness: A Multivariate Model of Residential Outcomes." *Rehabilitation Psychology*, 1993, *38* (4), 261–274.

Cook, J. A., and Razzano, L. "Followup Outcomes of Mothers Project Participants." Unpublished paper, Thresholds National Research and Training Center, Chicago, 1995.

Cook, J. A., Solomon, M. L., Farrell, D., Koziel, M., and Jonikus, J. A. "Psychiatric Rehabilitation for Transition-Age Youth with Severe Mental Illness: Program Model and Client Outcomes." In S. H. Henggeler and A. Santos (eds.), *Innovative Services for Difficult to Treat Populations*. New York: American Psychiatric Press, in press.

Cook, J. A., Solomon, M. L., and Mock, L. O. "What Happens After the First Job Placement: Vocational Transitioning Among Severely Emotionally Disturbed and Behavior Disordered Adolescents." *Programming for Adolescents with Behavioral Disorders*, 1989, *4*, 71–93.

Cook, J. A., Urwin, S. J., and Osborne, S. A. *Thresholds Annual Report: Fiscal Year 1994.* Chicago: Thresholds National Research and Training Center, 1994.

Farrell, D. "Effects of a Wilderness Camping Experience on Emotionally Disturbed Adolescents: Self-Esteem, Closeness and Symptomatology." Unpublished master's thesis, Rehabilitation Institute in the Graduate School, Southern Illinois University, 1982.

Korr, W. S., and Joseph, A. "Housing the Homeless Mentally Ill: An Experimental Evaluation." Unpublished manuscript, Jane Addams College of Social Work, University of Illinois at Chicago, 1994.

Kozlowski-Graham, K. "Comprehensive Mental Health Services for Deaf People with Major Mental Illness." *Hospital and Community Psychiatry*, 1991.

Kozlowski-Graham, K., Cook, J. A., and Razzano, L. *Twelve Month Outcomes of Deaf Clients with Severe Mental Illness Following Psychosocial Rehabilitation.* Chicago: Thresholds National Research and Training Center, 1995.

Lyons, J. S., Cook, J. A., Ruth, A., Karver, M., and Slagg, N. B. "Consumer Service Delivery in a Mobile Crisis Assessment Program." *Community Mental Health Journal*, in press.

Roussel, A. E., and Cook, J. A. "The Role of Work in Psychiatric Rehabilitation: The Visiting Chefs Program." *Sociological Practice*, 1987, *6*, 149–168.

Slagg, N. B., Lyons, J., Cook, J. A., Wasmer, D., and Ruth, A. "A Profile of Clients Served by a Mobile Outreach Program for Homeless Mentally Ill Persons." *Hospital and Community Psychiatry*, 1994, *45* (11), 1139–1141.

Stott, F. M., Musick, J. S., Cohler, B. J., Spencer, K. K., Goldman, J., Clark, R., and Dincin, J. "Intervention for the Severely Disturbed Mother." In B. J. Cohler and J. S. Musick (eds.), *Interventions Among Psychiatrically Impaired Parents and Their Young Children*. New Directions for Mental Health Services, no. 24. San Francisco: Jossey-Bass, 1984.

Task Force on Homelessness and Severe Mental Illness. *Outcasts on Main Street: Report of the Federal Task Force on Homelessness and Severe Mental Illness.* Washington, D.C.: Interagency Council on Homelessness, 1992.

Willerman, M., Wessell, M. E., and Cook, J. A. "The Effects of a Special Education Program on the Reading and Mathematics Achievement and Predictor Variables of a Severely Behavior Disabled Population." *Mid-Western Educational Researcher*, 1986, *8*, 42–43.

JERRY DINCIN is executive director of Thresholds.

MARY ANN ZEITZ is program director of the Thresholds Mothers Project.

DIANE FARRELL is program director of the Thresholds Young Adult Program.

LINDA HARRINGTON is program director of the Thresholds Program for Deaf and Mentally Ill Persons.

WALTER GREEN is program director of the Thresholds Short-Term Program for Homeless Mentally Ill Persons.

DEBBIE PAVICK is program director of the Thresholds Long-Term Program for Homeless Mentally Ill Persons.

CAMILLE RUCKS is program director of the Thresholds Program for Mentally Ill Substance Abusers.

PETER ILLING is program director of the Thresholds Older Adult Program.

Thresholds' degree of success in meeting its six program goals
has been consistently evaluated and researched for many years.

Program Evaluation and Research at Thresholds

Judith A. Cook

In 1978, the Schaffner Trust created the endowment that supports the Thresholds Research Institute and has enabled the agency to make an ongoing commitment to research. This commitment is twofold: first, to evaluate all components of the agency's programs by tracking the outcomes of all Thresholds members, and second, to conduct basic research on mental illness and psychiatric rehabilitation. The endowment supports ongoing evaluation of day-to-day service delivery in each of the agency's goal areas, while special time-limited grants from various federal agencies, the Illinois Department of Mental Health, and foundations fund special research projects. In October of 1990, the institute received a federal grant to establish the Thresholds National Research and Training Center on Rehabilitation and Mental Illness. While national in scope, the center has conducted several research projects at Thresholds that have added to the agency's repertoire of research knowledge.

This chapter takes a retrospective look at the research that has been conducted over the years at Thresholds. The intent is not to be exhaustive but illustrative and summative. In other words, studies are used to exemplify what the agency has learned about its programming and about the features of members who benefit most from receiving services. The chapter is organized around the six Thresholds goals, with special attention to studies examining the effectiveness of agency services and member outcomes.

Avoidance of Hospitalization

Numerous studies have illustrated that services members receive at Thresholds reduce member use of psychiatric inpatient services. In one study conducted

NEW DIRECTIONS FOR MENTAL HEALTH SERVICES, no. 68, Winter 1995 © Jossey-Bass Publishers

in the early 1980s, 102 members were randomly assigned to receive either Thresholds psychosocial rehabilitation (PSR) day program services or a peer support group (Dincin and Witheridge, 1982). At the end of a nine-month period of service delivery, Thresholds members had a 14 percent hospitalization rate, compared with 44 percent for control group members. While Thresholds members averaged 7.4 days of psychiatric hospitalization, the control group averaged a significantly higher 46.7 days. PSR services were clearly superior to peer support in helping members limit their use of psychiatric inpatient services.

Another study compared the effectiveness of assertive community treatment (ACT) services delivered by the Thresholds Bridge program with that of a readily accessible, low-expectation drop-in (DI) center (Bond and others, 1990). Eighty-eight members, averaging over seventeen lifetime psychiatric hospitalizations each, were randomly assigned to the two conditions and followed for twelve months. During the treatment year, ACT members had significantly fewer episodes of state hospitalization (1.2) than did DI members (2.6). Similarly, ACT members had significantly fewer days of state hospitalization (26.1) than did DI members (54.4). Moreover, the ACT group had a significant reduction of hospital episodes and hospital days compared to the preceding year, whereas the DI group did not. Thus, Thresholds' ACT model helped members reduce their use of inpatient services over time and did so more effectively than the DI model.

Research has indicated that ACT services have a significant catchment area impact on hospitalization. This was shown by a study designed to determine whether use of inpatient services at a state hospital was reduced by implementation of an ACT program in one of the hospital's catchment areas for members who were at especially high risk for hospitalization (Dincin and others, 1993). Bed-day utilization by sixty-six program participants during the fiscal year before the program was implemented (1986) was compared to the three subsequent fiscal years and to utilization rates of catchment areas not served by the program. Utilization of bed-days by persons in the ACT program's catchment area was reduced by 28 percent in the third fiscal year after program implementation, compared with an increase of 15 percent among persons in the hospital's other catchment areas. In the year after the program was implemented, participants were hospitalized for a mean of twenty-eight days, compared with a mean of eighty days in the year before the program. This study showed that the assertive community treatment program significantly reduced use of inpatient days and improved continuity of care.

Other research has explored such related topics as the ongoing proportion of Thresholds members hospitalized across multiple fiscal years. Data from the institute's annual reports (Cook, Urwin, and Osborne, 1994) indicate that over the past nine fiscal years, the percentage of members hospitalized has varied from 18 percent to 24 percent of all members served in psychosocial rehabilitation day programs and from 21 percent to 36 percent of all those in ACT programs. A study of 252 hospitalization incidents over a thirty-month period

(Jusko, 1987) to examine the reasons why members were hospitalized indicated that many contributing factors were nonpsychiatric. They included such problems as inadequate housing, failure of professionals to communicate effectively with Thresholds staff, poor discharge planning on the part of hospital staff, family conflict, and system-level constraints.

For the past ten years, Thresholds case managers have completed a brief questionnaire each time a hospitalization has occurred among the members on their caseload. The resulting information has allowed us to compare the proportion of all member hospitalizations involving medication nonadherence, with nonadherence defined as taking too much or too little medication, not taking prescribed medication at all, or fluctuating between taking too much and too little. At Thresholds North, the proportion of hospitalizations involving nonadherence has varied over the past ten years from a low of 30 percent to a high of 45 percent. Clearly, medication nonadherence is involved in a significant proportion of hospitalizations, and these findings have been incorporated into the planning of Thresholds programming in order to maximize agency effectiveness in helping members avoid unnecessary psychiatric hospitalizations.

Vocational Rehabilitation

Several studies indicate that members who receive Thresholds vocational services find jobs in the community. This has been demonstrated in randomized-design studies, in longitudinal research, and in annual report summaries.

In the United States as a whole, the employment rate among former psychiatric patients has been estimated at approximately 10 to 20 percent (Anthony, Cohen, and Vitalo, 1978; Frey, 1994). In contrast, the employment rate among Thresholds members while they are receiving vocational services varies from 50 percent to 80 percent (Cook and Razzano, 1993).

According to extensive employment data gathered over a seven-year period, the percentage of the active day program members at Thresholds who were gainfully employed has varied between 45 percent and 55 percent of all enrolled members. Correspondingly, the intake data for each of these years show that the percentage of members employed at time of entry into the program ranged from 3 percent to 7 percent. Estimating conservatively, this represents an increase of 40 percentage points in the proportion employed. Moreover, a study of all day program members employed over a six and one-half year period showed that they were working an average of 61 percent of their total time open in the program (Cook and Razzano, 1995). Thus, Thresholds programming increases the proportion of members who are working and keeps them employed for roughly two-thirds of the time they receive services from the agency.

Follow-up data gathered six months after members' termination from one of the Thresholds day programs over the past six years indicate that the percentage employed since termination has ranged from 34 percent to 45 percent.

Not surprisingly, the percentage employed at the time of the follow-up interview is somewhat lower, ranging from 23 percent to 35 percent. In a combined data set including ex-members followed up over a six-year period, the average hourly salary among those employed was $3.90, and the average number of hours worked weekly was twenty-one. Thus, even after leaving the agency, a noteworthy proportion of members are able to maintain the vocational gains they made while at Thresholds.

Another study examined job leaving over a thirty-six month period among 326 members, 74 youths and 252 adults, who worked between July 1986 and June 1989 (Cook, 1994). Data from 627 job endings indicated that youths and their adult counterparts had similar tenures on agency-sponsored placements but significantly different tenures on independent jobs. While adults held their independent jobs for an average of seven months, youths averaged only three months. Youths also were significantly more likely than adults to be fired from both placements and independent jobs; on independent jobs, the proportion of firings for youths (44 percent) was more than twice that for adults (19 percent). When reasons for job ending were examined, youths were more likely to lose jobs owing to aggressive or uncooperative behavior, while adults were more likely to end jobs owing to concentration difficulties and problems performing job tasks. These results support the need of young workers for jobs with more supervision and structure than adults require, and also indicate that adults will benefit from positions allowing on-site supports for training and reassurance.

Another study looked at program activities that predicted employment outcomes once members had left the agency (Cook and Rosenberg, 1994). Participants in the study were 448 ex-members of Thresholds interviewed six months after they left the program. The study found that the employed ex-members were those who had worked independently during their participation in the program or who had worked first on job-training placements and then their own jobs, compared to those ex-members who had never worked outside the agency or had worked only at agency-sponsored placements. In addition, ex-members who received continuous agency support after completing the vocational rehabilitation program were more likely to be working than those who terminated services completely or received intermittent support. The findings from this research point to the importance of members' gaining experience in the competitive labor market and receiving continual vocational support in maintaining employment at follow-up.

Several research studies conducted at Thresholds concern the use of vocational assessment to measure work behaviors and attitudes and plan vocational support services. Three studies have evaluated situational assessment, a hallmark of the Thresholds vocational approach. In one study, the situational assessment method used by Thresholds was used to predict employment outcomes for seventy-seven members followed up after fifteen months (Bond and Friedmeyer, 1987). The assessment form was a twenty-two-item checklist comprising four dimensions: work readiness, work attitudes, interpersonal relations, and work quality. Ratings were made in two work settings: prevocational work crews and transitional employment placements. Staff ratings made in both settings were predictive of later employment outcomes and predicted employment status better than did work history. In another study of the work histories of one hundred consecutive intakes at Thresholds (Cook and Engstrom, 1985), the last situational assessment before the member's first job was predictive of such vocational indicators as ability to achieve group and individual placements as well as independent employment, total number of positions held, and number of jobs in each type of position. Moreover, when compared with the predictive value of such other features as member demographics, work history, and illness features, the crew evaluations were more strongly related to vocational outcomes. The situational assessment also predicted employment and hourly salaries at six months and twelve months after assessment in a group of seventy-eight youths with mental illness (Cook and Weakland, 1991).

In another study, Bond and Dincin (1986) compared two randomly assigned groups of new members. One group participated in standard prevocational crew experiences at the agency for at least four months prior to being eligible for paid vocational placements outside the agency. An "accelerated" group was assigned to paid placements (conducted on a small-group basis) one month after intake. After fifteen months, 20 percent of the accelerated subjects were in competitive employment, compared with 7 percent of gradual subjects ($p < .10$), and only 15 percent of accelerated subjects were in prevocational crews, compared with 35 percent of gradual subjects ($p < .02$). All seven of the members working full-time at fifteen months were in the accelerated group. Work-experienced subjects benefited the most from the accelerated approach. There were no differences between conditions in rehospitalization rates. The results of this study suggest that shortening the prevocational preparation period can benefit some members, particularly those with prior work experience.

Residential Rehabilitation

Research has examined the effectiveness of Thresholds services in helping members live independently (that is, in their own homes or apartments) in the community. For example, longitudinal data for one group of 650 ex-members of Thresholds day programming showed that the percentage living in their own apartments or houses rose from 15 percent at time of program entry to 36 percent at time of termination, and remained at 34 percent six months later at follow-up (Cook, 1994). Multivariate statistical analysis indicated that those ex-members who were living independently at follow-up had significantly higher levels of functioning, had participated in Thresholds significantly longer, were more likely to be parents, had higher community participation levels, and were less likely to be receiving ongoing agency services. Notably, this study found no significant relationship between use of the Thresholds housing program and better residential outcomes. This was not the case in a study that looked at the residential and vocational outcomes of only those members who were working at the six-month follow-up (Cook and Razzano, 1993). This latter study of 166 ex-members found that those who had lived in Thresholds housing were more likely to be successful both residentially and vocationally or to be successful residentially but not vocationally, while those who had not participated in the housing program were more likely to be either unsuccessful both residentially and vocationally or to be successful vocationally but not residentially.

In another study of sixty assertive outreach members who were deaf or hearing impaired (Cook, Kozlowski-Graham, and Razzano, 1993), the percentage living in their own apartments and houses rose from 20 percent at the time of program entry to 45 percent while they were in the program. Multivariate analysis revealed that those more likely to live on their own were higher functioning, were younger at their first psychiatric treatment, were more likely to be Caucasian than minority, were more likely to have a diagnosis of schizophrenia, and were more likely to have a history of competitive employment.

Earlier program evaluation studies conducted in fiscal years 1975–76 (Dincin and Kaberon, 1979) and 1982–83 (Mirsky, 1983) illustrate a movement toward more independent living arrangements. Mirsky's study looked retrospectively at changes in living arrangements for 220 active members, half of whom had attended for more than twelve months. Dincin and Kaberon examined changes at closing for 153 members who had averaged ten and one-half months of attendance. In the 1975–76 study, the percentage living independently increased from 24 percent at intake to 39 percent at closing. There was a corresponding decrease in the percentage living with parents, from 38 percent at intake to 23 percent at closing. In the 1982–83 study, the percentage living independently increased from 18 percent to 28 percent and the percentage living with parents decreased from 47 percent to 26 percent. Altogether, 48 percent of the current Thresholds membership in this latter study were living more independently than at intake, 46 percent were living at the same level, and only 6 percent were living less independently.

Educational Rehabilitation

Several studies conducted at Thresholds have documented members' needs for remedial education when they enter the agency. One study of math and reading skills among 248 incoming members (Cook, Wessell, and Dincin, 1987) found an average score of grade 8 for mathematical computation and grade 9 for reading comprehension, despite the fact that the mean number of years of education for this group was twelve years. Over half (55 percent) of all incoming members scored below grade 10 in reading while over three-quarters (77 percent) did so in mathematics. Even among a group of members selected to receive postsecondary educational services, large academic deficits were found. A Wide Range Achievement Test (Jastak and Wilkinson, 1984) screening of ninety-six members entering the transition-to-college program (CSP) at Thresholds (Cook and Solomon, 1993) indicated that one-third (34 percent) performed math below grade 12 level and 27 percent performed below grade 8, while a quarter (25 percent) read below grade 12 level and 13 percent read below grade 8. Clearly, large numbers of members entering the agency need help improving educational skills.

The effectiveness of Thresholds remedial educational services was demonstrated in one study of sixty-five youths with severe mental illness participating in the Thresholds accredited high school program (Willerman, Wessell, and Cook, 1986). Following one hundred hours of instruction, their scores increased significantly on both reading and mathematics. Moreover, while students' age, ethnicity, gender, and parental marital status were related to their math and reading scores when they began the program, these variables were not related to their scores following one hundred hours of instruction. An earlier study of thirty-seven consecutive students completing one hundred hours of instruction toward their high school diplomas revealed average pretest/posttest gains of 1.3 grade levels in reading and 1.5 levels in mathematics (Bond, Dincin, Setze, and Witheridge, 1984). These results suggest that those receiving secondary educational services show significant gains over time and that educational services may override the effects of students' demographic and familial features.

Research also has examined the effectiveness of Thresholds postsecondary educational services. One study of 125 members who participated in the three-year transition-to-college program called the Community Scholars Program (Cook and Solomon, 1993) found that 42 percent had taken at least one mainstream class at a college, university, or trade school; the average number of courses completed (for example, for which a final grade was received) was 3.6. During the same time, 78 percent of all students held at least one job, with 47 percent of all former members employed at the time of their follow-up interview. Paired t tests indicated statistically significant increases in ex-members' hourly salaries and in the number of hours they were employed per week after participating in the program. In addition to significant educational and vocational gains, the study also found significant increases in participants' self-esteem and coping mastery after participating in the program. Interestingly, these increases were not accompanied by increases in anxiety, showing that the program may have helped members deal with the stresses associated with attending college or trade school.

A medication education program for Thresholds members was evaluated in another study in which forty members were randomly assigned to an education group and thirty-five to a control group (Streicker, Amdur, and Dincin, 1986). Pretesting, posttesting, and follow-up testing of medication compliance, medication attitudes, and medication knowledge were conducted. Results indicated that the medication education group significantly improved members' knowledge about psychotropic drugs and that this information was retained at follow-up. However, while attitudes towards medication improved at posttesting, they worsened at follow-up, while medication compliance was significantly worse in the experimental group than among the control subjects at both posttesting and follow-up. Thus, while this type of education significantly improves knowledge about medications, it has less impact on attitudes toward taking medication and no positive impact on adherence to medication regimens.

Social Rehabilitation

Studies have examined the effects of many of the social and leisure activities engaged in by Thresholds members, both those resulting from activities sponsored by the agency and from members' more independent use of community resources. Several years of follow-up research has examined the social and leisure time activities of members six months after they leave the day program. These studies use the Leisure Time Activities Scale of Katz and Lyerly (1963), which asks about the frequency with which individuals engage in socializing (visiting friends, visiting family, entertaining friends), community participation activities (clubs, sports, religious activities), and solitary activities (watching television, listening to the radio, sleeping during the daytime). One report on 109 ex-members at six-month follow-up indicated that they engaged in an average of seven out of the fourteen social and community participation activities on the Leisure Time Activities Scale (Razzano and Gervain, 1990). Thus, even after members leave the agency, they continue to engage in a noteworthy amount of community participation and socializing.

The agency's therapeutic camping program was the focus of one quasi-experimental study designed to assess its effectiveness on a group of thirteen youths with severe mental illness (Farrell, 1982). The thirteen youths who attended camp were compared to a quasi–control group comprising nine youths not attending camp. Measures of self-esteem, cohesiveness, and symptomatology were taken at three points: two weeks prior to camp, the last day of camp (for the campers) or the first day of agency reopening (for the quasi–control group), and one month after the completion of camp. Results indicated that campers experienced enhanced self-esteem, increased feelings of closeness, and diminished symptomatology while the comparison group did not. However, self-esteem was the sole effect to remain significant at follow-up, suggesting that the camping program's positive effects were limited in duration.

Promotion of Physical Health and Well-Being

The 1987 addition of the Thresholds goal of promoting physical health and well-being inaugurated attention to the effectiveness of agency services in this area. While much less research has been done here compared to the other goal areas, one completed study has examined Thresholds HIV prevention services. The study examined an agencywide HIV risk factor assessment and testing project conducted in 1994 as part of a general health promotion campaign.

This project screened 757 Thresholds members (Cook, Razzano, and others, 1994). Fifty-one percent reported one or more of the following risk factors: intravenous (IV) drug use, sex with an IV drug user, male homosexual sex, sex with a bisexual man, history of STDs, recreational drug use, alcohol use, and receipt of a blood transfusion prior to 1985. When alcohol use is excluded, this proportion falls to 39 percent; when both alcohol and non-IV drug use are excluded, the proportion is still about a third (35 percent). In addition, 39 percent (295 members) said they were sexually active, yet 26 percent said they "never" used condoms, and another 36 percent reported less than faithful condom usage. Since the intent of the screening was to identify those members suitable for HIV antibody testing, the study examined whether or not those members identified as at risk by the assessment subsequently were recommended by their caseworkers for testing. Results revealed that this did indeed occur, even when controlling for the effects of members' age group (adolescent versus adult), ethnicity (Caucasian versus minority), locale (rural versus urban), or service model (ACT versus PSR day program). Thus, staff used the screening instrument appropriately in making HIV test recommendations. Unfortunately, data regarding whether or not members followed caseworkers' recommendations are not available.

Overview of Agency Effectiveness

This review of research conducted at Thresholds over the years since the agency's inception illustrates many aspects of the agency's effectiveness. Additional studies of the agency exist, many of which are mentioned in this volume in sections on specific programs, such as those tailored for youths, mothers, homeless individuals, and deaf persons with severe mental illness. Still other studies have been conducted on topics such as family coping with adult offspring who have mental illness, cost effectiveness of the agency's services, and correlates of program attrition. An *Annotated Bibliography of Research at Thresholds* (Cook, Roussel, Straiton, and Goode, 1993), which includes all these studies, can be obtained by contacting the agency. The following paragraphs summarize the results illustrated in the foregoing review of studies relating to the six Thresholds goals.

First, Thresholds programs reduce hospitalizations, both their number and their length. In addition, a low proportion of members are hospitalized during the time they are actively involved in programming, and this low rate has been maintained by the various agency programs for over a decade. Second, Thresholds helps people prepare for, obtain, and maintain community employment, although those who terminate services completely have poorer outcomes than those whose vocational support is uninterrupted. Third, the proportion of members living in commercially available housing rises over time with service delivery, suggesting that the program improves members' levels of independent living. Members' needs for remedial education have been clearly demonstrated by agency research, as has members' ability to benefit from supported education in attending high school, college, or trade school. The participation of members in community activities and in socializing with friends and family continues even after ending services. Finally, physical health screenings including HIV test recommendations to members were effective in reaching those who were at-risk for HIV infection according to self-reported risk factors.

The value of research conducted in service delivery settings is illustrated throughout this chapter. Such research is better able than academic or laboratory research to address service delivery issues of direct relevance to staff and members. An additional advantage is that the results of such studies can then be used to alter or enhance programming in the very settings in which the research occurred. The commitment to research and evaluation made many years ago at Thresholds has served the agency well in the past and will help guide the agency into the twenty-first century.

References

Anthony, W. A., Cohen, M. R., and Vitalo, R. "The Measurement of Rehabilitation Outcome." *Schizophrenia Bulletin*, 1978, *4*, 365–383.

Bond, G. R., and Dincin, J. "Accelerating Entry into Transitional Employment in a Psychosocial Rehabilitation Agency." *Rehabilitation Psychology*, 1986, *31*, 143–155.

Bond, G. R., Dincin, J., Setze, P. J., and Witheridge, T. F. "The Effectiveness of Psychiatric Rehabilitation: A Summary of Research at Thresholds." *Psychosocial Rehabilitation Journal*, 1984, *7*, 6–22.

Bond, G. R., and Friedmeyer, M. H. "Predictive Validity of Situational Assessment at a Psychiatric Rehabilitation Center." *Rehabilitation Psychology*, 1987, *32*, 99–112.

Bond, G. R., Witheridge, T. F., Dincin, J., Wasmer, D., Webb, J., and De Graaf-Kaiser, R. "Assertive Community Treatment for Frequent Users of Psychiatric Hospitals in a Large City: A Controlled Study." *American Journal of Community Psychology*, 1990, *18*, 865–891.

Cook, J. A. "Independent Community Living Among Women with Severe Mental Illness: A Comparison with Outcomes Among Men." *Journal of Mental Health Administration*, 1994, *21* (4), 361–373.

Cook, J. A., and Engstrom, K. "Using Prevocational Crew Ratings on the Thresholds' Work Reporting Form to Predict Later Client Employment (Research Note #17)." Chicago: Thresholds Research Institute, 1985.

Cook, J. A., Kozlowski-Graham, K., and Razzano, L. "Psychosocial Rehabilitation of Deaf Persons with Severe Mental Illness: A Multivariate Model of Residential Outcomes." *Rehabilitation Psychology*, 1993, *38* (4), 261–274.

Cook, J. A., and Razzano, L. "Natural Vocational Supports for Persons with Severe Mental Illness: Thresholds Supported Competitive Employment Program." In L. I. Stein (ed.), *Innovative Community Mental Health Programs*. New Directions for Mental Health Services, no. 56. San Francisco: Jossey-Bass, 1992.

Cook, J. A., and Razzano, L. "A Canonical Correlation Analysis of Vocational and Residential Outcomes in a Multidimensional Psychiatric Rehabilitation Program." Paper presented at the annual conference of the American Sociological Association, Miami, Fla., 1993.

Cook, J. A., and Razzano, L. "Discriminant Function Analysis of Competitive Employment Outcomes in a Transitional Employment Program for Persons with Severe Mental Illness." *Journal of Vocational Rehabilitation*, 1995, *5*, 127–139.

Cook, J. A., Razzano, L., Jayaraj, A., Myers, M. K., Nathanson, F., Stott, M. A., and Stein, M. "HIV Risk Assessment for Psychiatric Rehabilitation Clientele: Implications for Community-Based Services." *Psychosocial Rehabilitation Journal,* 1994, *17* (4), 105–116.

Cook, J. A., and Rosenberg, H. "Predicting Community Employment Among Persons with Psychiatric Disability: A Logistic Regression Analysis." *Journal of Rehabilitation Administration,* 1994, *18* (1), 6–22.

Cook, J. A., Roussel, A. E., Straiton, D. M., and Goode, S. *Annotated Bibliography of Research at Thresholds.* Chicago: Thresholds Research Institute, 1993.

Cook, J. A., and Solomon, M. L. "The Community Scholar Program: An Outcome Study of Supported Education for Students with Severe Mental Illness." *Psychosocial Rehabilitation Journal,* 1993, *17* (1), 83–97.

Cook, J. A., Urwin, S. J., and Osborne, S. A. *Thresholds Annual Report: Fiscal Year 1994.* Chicago: Thresholds National Research and Training Center, 1994.

Cook, J. A., and Weakland, R. "Vocational Rehabilitation for Youth with Severe Mental Illness: Predictive Validity of Situational Assessment for Later Employment." Paper presented at the 119th annual meeting of the American Public Health Association, Atlanta, 1991.

Cook, J. A., Wessell, M. E., and Dincin, J. "Predicting Educational Achievement Levels of the Severely Mentally Ill: Implications for the Psychosocial Program Administrator." *Psychosocial Rehabilitation Journal,* 1987, *11* (1), 23–37.

Dincin, J., and Kaberon, D. A. *Attendance as a Predictor of Success in Rehabilitation of Former Psychiatric Patients: Final Report to the Chicago Community Trust.* Chicago: Thresholds Research Institute, 1979.

Dincin, J., and Witheridge, T. F. "Psychiatric Rehabilitation as a Deterrent to Recidivism." *Hospital and Community Psychiatry,* 1982, *33,* 645–650.

Dincin, J., Witheridge, T. F., Wasmer, D., Sobeck, L., Cook, J. A., and Razzano, L. "The Impact of Assertive Community Treatment on Hospital Utilization in an Urban Catchment Area." *Hospital and Community Psychiatry,* 1993, *44* (9), 833–838.

Farrell, D. "Effects of a Wilderness Camping Experience on Emotionally Disturbed Adolescents: Self-Esteem, Closeness and Symptomatology." Unpublished master's thesis, Rehabilitation Administration and Services Graduate School, Southern Illinois University, 1982.

Frey, J. L. "Long Term Support: The Critical Element to Sustaining Competitive Employment: Where Do We Begin?" *Psychosocial Rehabilitation Journal,* 1994, *17* (3), 127–134.

Jastak, S., and Wilkinson, G. S. *Wide Range Achievement Test: Level 2.* Wilmington: Jastak Associates, 1984.

Jusko, R. A. "A Descriptive Analysis of Factors in Psychiatric Readmission." Unpublished master's thesis, Social Sciences Division, University of Chicago, 1987.

Katz, M. M., and Lyerly, S. B. "Methods for Measuring Adjustment and Social Behavior in the Community. I: Rationale, Description, Discriminative Validity, and Scale Development." *Psychological Reports,* 1963, *13,* 503–535.

Mirsky, K. *Thresholds Members' Residence: Descriptive Report.* Chicago: Thresholds Research Institute, 1983.

Razzano, L., and Gervain, M. *Thresholds Research Institute Follow-Up Report: Fiscal Year 1990.* Chicago: Thresholds National Research and Training Center, 1990.

Streicker, S. K., Amdur, M., and Dincin, J. "Educating Patients About Psychiatric Medications: Failure to Enhance Compliance." *Psychosocial Rehabilitation Journal,* 1986, *9,* 15–28.

Willerman, M., Wessell, M. E., and Cook, J. A. "The Effects of a Special Education Program on the Reading and Mathematics Achievement and Predictor Variables of a Severely Behavior Disabled Population." *Mid-Western Educational Researcher,* 1986, *8,* 42–43.

JUDITH A. COOK is director of Thresholds National Research and Training Center.

A strong organizational and decentralized administrative philosophy
is the underpinning of growth, program development, and quality.

Organizational Issues

Jerry Dincin

There is a lot more to operating an organization such as Thresholds than the work directly with members themselves. A structure to support the frontline work and, most importantly, the development of a board of directors to help guide the organization must be established and nurtured. Beside the development of a supportive board, an agency also has to learn to deal with finances in a professional manner.

Board of Directors

From the very beginning, the Thresholds board has been a huge asset. There are several areas of board functioning that require any agency's attention.

Board Development. The role of the Thresholds board of directors has grown from an advisory one to a much more expanded responsibility, especially in the areas of financial oversight and policy making. In the beginning years, the board was perhaps overly involved with the program, leading to confusion and an inability on the part of the professional staff to define their role. That issue changed dramatically in 1965 when I was hired (becoming the young agency's fifth executive director). The board understood from that point on that the executive director was in charge of program operations while the board was to set basic policy and direction.

It is important to have ongoing discussion of the responsibilities of board members, and at Thresholds, we review this issue periodically. The following document, entitled "What Does an Effective Board Member Do?" has been adopted as board policy.

1. An effective Board Member takes the opportunity and responsibility to familiarize him/herself with the theory and practices of the Thresholds Program for rehabilitating the mentally ill.

2. An effective Board Member makes an active commitment to
    a. Help decide basic policy questions
    b. Oversee financial aspects of the agency
    c. Work as a public relations advocate
    d. Seek employment for members
    e. Search out appropriate volunteers
    f. Participate in Long Range Planning.
3. An effective Board Member assumes these significant financial and fund raising responsibilities:
    a. Gives a yearly financial contribution for operational expenses at a level that comfortably expresses their financial resources and their interest and commitment to Thresholds.
    b. Supports and participates in the Board's major fund raising events (benefits) by attending, approaching friends to attend, and assisting in some aspect of the event.
    c. Develops a list of fund raising prospects (individuals, foundations, and corporations) that he/she will solicit for Thresholds in order to raise at least $1,000 from the community. Solicitations are usually in the form of a letter and it is suggested that each Board Member send out at least 15 letters.
    d. Considers a possibility of a deferred gift.
4. An effective Board Member serves on at least one committee and attends a majority of the Board Meetings.
5. An effective Board Member recommends new Board Members for nomination.
6. An effective Board Member attends Board Retreats.
7. An effective Board Member gives Thresholds a high priority on his/her list of charitable giving.

Board Functioning. Our board functions on a committee system. The executive committee meets monthly. The entire board meets nine times a year.

One indication of board interest and commitment is the longevity of board members. On our board, all of the living past presidents remain on the board, and several board members have served since the beginning, making for experienced participation. (Board members serve two-year terms.)

Five-Year Plans. The board charts a general course for Thresholds through five-year plans. The executive director drafts the five-year plan with input from senior and line staff, members, and members' families, outlining the areas he would like to see emphasized in the coming years. A board committee reviews the recommendations in the draft and makes additions and deletions. Almost six months is spent on plan evaluation before the plan is adopted by the board.

The five-year plan is intended to chart the general direction for agency programs without locking the agency into any single goal or strategy. It is not a blueprint but a guide. Our five-year plan helps us to make a full-court press on whatever the plan commits us to, but we are not limited to working on areas delineated in the plan. When promising opportunities arise, the agency and the board can decide to move in a new direction. The board also reexamines the agency mission statement periodically, to update or revise it when necessary. In the Thresholds mission statement, the agency commits to these actions:

1. To provide a broad range of rehabilitation recovery and partial hospitalization services in the community for persons with mental illness, for as long as they are needed.
2. To develop new services and expand existing services to help meet the needs of our members and to improve the quality of life of a wide range of persons with severe and persistent mental illness. Quality of life includes prevention of unnecessary hospitalization; vocational rehabilitation, social rehabilitation, education, and independent living; physical health and well-being.
3. To evaluate the results of our efforts through research and disseminate them through training, consultation, publications, and conference presentations.
4. To address the stigma of mental illness and to change the climate of acceptance for persons with mental illness.
5. To develop demonstration projects as prototypes for treatment, evaluation, or rehabilitation approaches.

Board Concerns. Obviously, a board has its own unique concerns. Some of them at Thresholds, especially in the beginning, had to do with taking bolder steps into new programs. The board and executive director have a mutual respect for each other's abilities and a mutual commitment that has deepened over the years. One of the greatest strengths of our board is its ability to offer an outside perspective, particularly in business matters affecting the agency.

Board presidents are also central to the success of an agency through their leadership at times of uncertainty or expansion. Their understanding acceptance of the difference between the policy and fundraising role of the board president and the operational role of the executive director, makes for a smooth running team with mutual trust at its core. There are very few board members who actually enjoy the task of asking their friends and acquaintances for money, and it must be the role modeling and constant emphasis of the president that makes this task a prime recognized responsibility. The president must promote it with energy and conviction. At Thresholds, the finding of job placements for members and the development of housing have similarly been spearheaded by knowledgeable board members, particularly the president. Much is owed to our group of men and women who have served in this role. Each deserves the grateful appreciation of staff, members, and the mental health community for having given so much as volunteers to a stigmatized and neglected group of clientele.

Fundraising. It has taken many years for the board, together with our development office, to learn how to raise significant sums from community sources. Our fundraising occurs through board members' personal gifts and the contributions they solicit from their friends, through foundation and corporate gifts, and through fundraising benefits. The largest benefit event at Thresholds is our annual Golf and Tennis Benefit, held at a North Shore country club. The first such outing, in 1986, netted $25,000; the 1994 outing netted $150,000. In fiscal 1994, board members and the development office raised over $1 million, which represents a very successful fundraising year for us. That sum does not include about $500,000 in one-time endowment gifts that were also brought in by the board.

In addition to its contributions to operations and endowments, the Thresholds board has been willing to take on special capital projects such as the purchase and renovation of our main headquarters' building. We were at a nexus in 1972 when the mansion in question became available. To us, $170,000 to purchase that building seemed like a huge sum of money. We also needed $350,000 for renovations. It was a moment of decision, and it was the board, led by Loren Juhl, that said, "Let's do it." Many thought the $5,000 earnest money was thrown away. Our latest major capital project, the purchase and renovation of the building for the Young Adult Program, raised $2 million. Board member contributions have also made it possible to purchase two group homes.

Board members' fundraising efforts with the support of our development office have made possible new programs, less dependence on government monies, and higher salary levels. The Thresholds board is a major factor in the solidity of the agency.

Program Organization

Thresholds program sites are spread out geographically. Although the bulk of the programs are located in Chicago, at their furthest point, Thresholds programs are one hundred miles apart. Thus, the agency has evolved a decentralized system, with program directors having local control while centralized issues are supervised by three assistant directors and an associate director, who meet with the executive director weekly along with the chief financial officer, comptroller, research director, and assistant to the executive director. Minutes of these meetings are distributed to all program directors.

We find it essential that program directors feel free to operate their programs, within the parameters of the six Thresholds goals and our funding constraints. There is plenty of room for them to adjust to local conditions and make necessary program accommodations for their particular clientele. For instance, Thresholds can accommodate both a fairly intensive psychotherapy program for older adolescents and assertive community treatment offices where almost no psychotherapy is offered. This difference demonstrates our respect for individual program direction at the local site, within the context of overall supervisory input by the most senior staff (who have an average agency tenure of fifteen years). The constant tension between the necessity of centralization in some areas (budget and fiscal control, standards for personnel, and documentation of member records) and the independent functioning of daily operations under local program directors has turned out to be a healthy tension.

The program directors for each site are responsible for developing proposed budgets, based on certain funding and salary assumptions. The proposed budget for each fiscal year is projected on the first nine months of the previous fiscal year. Each program director has to justify any additions or deletions to programming in a process that is extremely detailed. Monthly expense and revenue printouts tell program directors exactly where they stand in relation to budget.

Each program area is expected to be in the black. Program directors take this very seriously, and they should. In some cases, programs are in the black by only a very narrow margin, and the fact that they are on the black not the red side of our accounts illustrates the value of moving the locus of control into the program area. The program directors are truly responsible for program development and budget control. Unfortunately, despite our best efforts, as the agency has grown larger, more and more bureaucratic demands from headquarters, accrediting agencies, and funding sources are falling on the program directors.

Staff Training

Thresholds is reflecting the current general business interest in staff training. We now have 1.5 FTE staff positions devoted to in-service training with additional help on the way. In the past, staff training was informal and on the job. However, staff training performed in that way tends to get sloppy and disorganized. Now our training is divided into an orientation phase that continues through the three-month probation period, ongoing psychiatric rehabilitation training for line staff, and managerial training for supervisors. We are seriously addressing the problem of training residential staff, especially weekend staff and job coaches.

Diversity of staff training is extremely important. This is illustrated by the quantity and variety of staff training presentations in 1994. Some sixty-seven different presentations were given, and the following sample titles suggest their range: "Affective Disorders," "Basic MISA Training," "Basic Psychopharmacology," "Charting in Treatment Plans," "Clubhouse Model Comes of Age," "Corporations Make Great Partners," "Dysfunctional Families," "Federal Grants," "How to Manage Disruptive Behavior," "How to Do Mental Status Exams," "New Procedures for Med Monitoring," "Physical Defense," "Schizophrenia and Suicide," "Sociolinguistics of the Deaf Community," "Spirituality," and "Working with Members Around Sexuality."

In the future, staff training will be even more important for all agencies. At Thresholds, we will be expending more effort in this area, too, particularly on the topic of medication and side effects. Training money is money wisely invested.

Growth

Thresholds has grown by developing new branches, expanding its programs, and seeking diverse sources of funding.

Development of Branches. It has always been true that Thresholds wanted to have a larger impact on the mental health scene than could be contained in one location. Starting in 1968 with a foundation grant and VISTA workers, Thresholds opened its first branch in the ghetto of psychiatric patients that had emerged in the uptown area of Chicago. Since then, we have continually spread our services, to the south side of Chicago, to the rural area of Kankakee, and to various underserved areas of Chicago, contributing to both agency growth and the development of a statewide model for psychiatric rehabilitation.

Our partnership affiliation with local chapters of Alliance for the Mentally Ill (AMI) in the development of branches is another example of how agencies can grow successfully. We had become aware of the many problems that plagued programs operated directly by parents of the mentally ill. Many of these projects came apart at the seams after a few years. Yet parents needed input into the rehabilitation programs and a sense of ownership. In most mental health agencies and hospitals, they were treated poorly, without respect. Their needs and knowledge were rarely taken into account.

Thresholds engaged one suburban chapter of AMI in a cooperative arrangement wherein the chapter became a DMH grantee and then subcontracted program operation to Thresholds, which took care of all member activities and fiscal accountability. We decide mutually on the array of services, taking into account the special needs of these parents' children and emphasizing the program aspects the parents felt were needed the most. This partnership has had its problems, but generally it works well. The parents have a sense of empowerment because they are providing the services, but they do not have all the responsibilities that go with practical program operation.

Thresholds feels that parental input is valuable, and true partnerships in several locales have emerged, enlarging the number and scope of services that Thresholds offers. Usually these projects start small, with budgets under $100,000, but sometimes, in the right growth cycle, they can become $1 million projects with a wide range of services. Presently, this type of project is thriving in several Chicago suburbs. It is a model that other AMI groups and psychiatric rehabilitation centers could emulate.

Program Growth. Growth of Thresholds programs has been consistent. We have never had a year of program or revenue shrinkage. In fiscal year 1995, Thresholds had eight program sites with revenues of over $1 million. We believe that there are six reasons for this amazing record.

First, Thresholds Bridge programs have been rightly seen by funding sources as a prime effective method of reducing hospitalization for severely ill psychiatric patients. From one small Bridge program have grown four large ones, with a total budget of $5,223,000. Second, the creation of niche programs

Table 7.1. Thresholds Operating Revenue and Growth Pattern

Fiscal Year	Total Revenue	Increase over Prior Year	
		Dollars	Percentage
1975	$509,000		
1976	660,000	$151,000	29.7 %
1977	1,160,000	500,000	75.8
1978	1,460,000	300,000	25.8
1979	1,785,000	325,000	22.3
1980	1,894,000	109,000	6.1
1981	2,020,000	126,000	6.7
1982	2,193,000	173,000	8.6
1983	2,388,000	195,000	8.9
1984	2,800,000	412,000	17.3
1985	3,530,000	730,000	26.1
1986	4,830,000	1,300,000	36.8
1987	5,850,000	1,020,000	21.1
1988	6,820,000	970,000	16.6
1989	8,225,000	1,405,000	20.6
1990	11,152,000	2,927,000	35.6
1991	14,246,000	3,366,000	30.2
1992	15,240,000	994,000	7.0
1993	16,230,000	990,000	6.0
1994	19,150,000	2,920,000	18.0

Note: Excludes Thresholds rehabilitation industries and HUD housing corporations. Includes endowment contributions.

Fiscal Year	Number of Staff
1977	53
1979	62
1989	246
1990	250
1991	316
1992	325
1993	330
1994	421

for special groups of members and their successful funding has promoted organizational diversity. Third, investment in evaluation and research to demonstrate the effectiveness of Thresholds programs has been a primary underpinning of agency growth. Fourth, the strong emphasis on housing development and the commitment to providing clean, decent housing for our members generated a much needed service that fueled expansion. Fifth, establishment of successful Thresholds businesses, with an emphasis on the bottom line, led to many jobs for members and revenues of $2 million. Sixth, decisions to establish branches, to decentralize, and to become a contractor for several AMI groups led to expansion and a series of partnership arrangements with parent groups that were mutually beneficial.

Growth and Finances. Thresholds grows with the addition of each new program and each new house. Including the funds for all its subsidiary corporations, Thresholds' budget for fiscal year 1995 was $23,468,000.

We have been able to cap our administrative costs at 15 percent of our budget; these costs include 1 percent of our budget each for research and fundraising.

The vast majority of our funds are governmental, with the Illinois Department of Mental Health providing 58 percent of the total budget. However, Thresholds could not grow, experiment, and/or demonstrate without community donations. Each psychiatric rehabilitation agency needs to find and develop its own diverse mix of funding sources. At Thresholds, we decided not to depend on one source but rather to work in several programmatic and experimental directions both to spread the risk and to increase the eclectic nature of our funding sources while our services stayed focused on one needy population, people with serious and persistent mental illness.

On the expense side, 72 percent of our income goes into personnel costs. This is as it should be because we are heavily committed to line staff. Thresholds salaries are not generous. The starting salary for a person with a bachelor's degree is $20,000 a year. A staff person with a master's degree starts at $25,000 a year. To help mitigate those low salaries, Thresholds has a tremendous benefit package. We pay the full cost of hospital health care insurance and dental care insurance for both the employees and their families. The cost of employee benefits amounts to 26 percent of salaries.

Table 7.1 depicts Thresholds growth over the past twenty years (not including the subsidiary corporations). Remarkably, several Thresholds branches today have greater revenues than the entire organization did as recently as ten years ago. The table confirms what the preceding chapters in this volume have been emphasizing, that a private nonprofit agency can play a major role in meeting the need for psychiatric rehabilitation programs for the severely and persistently mentally ill.

JERRY DINCIN *is executive director of Thresholds.*

An array of emerging issues in psychiatric rehabilitation do not get enough discussion.

Current Challenges

Jerry Dincin

There are a number of issues that affect the psychiatric rehabilitation of the mentally ill but that agencies rarely address directly. They run the gamut from the stigma of mental illness to members' spirituality, from employing members as staff to educating members' families. It is time for all of us to be more aware of the ways in which these issues, seemingly peripheral when we are trying to cope with members' serious and most distressing symptoms, can hinder us or assist us in helping our members. This chapter is a start on fostering that awareness.

Stigma

The news on our television sets and in our newspapers every day engulfs us with stereotypical attitudes about mental illness and the prejudices consequent upon those attitudes, showing us how much work is still ahead of us. The stigma attached to mental illness is still a major problem for the mentally ill themselves and for those who treat them.

From the old Hitchcock thriller *Psycho* to the recent thriller *The Silence of the Lambs*, a stereotype exists and persists in popular culture that people with mental illness are not only sick but dangerously violent and unpredictable. The image pops up everywhere, even in advertising and, more importantly, in everyday speech and beliefs. The stereotype feeds a stigma that is almost as debilitating as the terrible illness itself. But there is hope. While it is still harmful, the stigma attached to mental illness has changed and diminished enormously just in my lifetime.

What I mean by stigma is not only the perceived danger but the disgrace associated with people who have a mental illness. While it is true that some people with a mental illness display erratic and sometimes unpredictable behavior, the public forms opinions based only on these more visible attributes of the illness. Because of these symptoms, most people want to distance themselves from anyone with mental illness. Because of the difficulty of understanding mental illness, the disease has been separated in the public's mind from other chronic diseases, such as diabetes or the damage from a bad stroke. Because of the sense of irrationality in some people with mental illness, the public is afraid. Part of that fear, I suspect, comes because people do not know if mental illness will happen to them.

For all these reasons, there is a great deal of prejudice. In past years, the public also blamed the parents of the mentally ill, creating a feeling of shame in those parents, born somehow of their responsibility. That blaming also contributed greatly to the stigma, as parents and families attempted to hide family members with mental illness because of the reflection on the family. The shift from blaming parents to enlisting their help in their children's recovery has diminished their guilt and helped to reduce the stigma.

In the past several decades, the prejudice or stigma surrounding mental illness has lessened considerably. Medication, by far, is the most important reason for this. Medication controls symptoms. Without medication, there would not be any rehabilitation programs like Thresholds. Without medication, people would still be cooped up in massive mental hospitals. A biological explanation for mental illness is the first and the central tool in fighting the stigma of mental illness. As new medications target specific symptoms with fewer side effects, mental illness will become less treacherous and fearsome, and that result will reduce stigma still more. Scientific advances in the pursuit of a precise biological cause for mental illness, just like the advances made in pursuing the causes for illnesses like amyotrophic lateral sclerosis and cancer, increase our understanding of the illness dramatically and also lessen the stigma associated with it (Dincin, 1993).

Several recent laws now mandate more equitable treatment of psychiatric patients. The Federal Fair Housing Act put psychiatric patients under the protective umbrella of a powerful federal law, making it illegal to discriminate against psychiatric patients, and in the change from housing discrimination to a greater sense of housing fairness, we have made tremendous gains. It is still too early to tell what effect the Americans with Disabilities Act will have, but classifying mental illness with other disabilities should have a very salutary effect. With the help of these laws, we will continue our work against discrimination. But we must not forget that discrimination is not the same as stigma. Perhaps our most powerful tool in combating stigma would be public acknowledgement that persons with mental illness can work productively and succeed in the same ways as people without this illness. Therefore, we should encourage more public attention to our members' personal accomplishments and their success stories as businesspeople, as artists, as professionals, and as students and teachers.

The Prosumer Movement: Members as Staff

There is no question that certain members who have experienced a mental illness can be especially empathic and helpful to other members. At Thresholds, we have tried to find such people and to offer them part-time and full-time jobs as *prosumers,* a term combining the words "professional" and "consumer" and describing staff who have had experiences as patients in the mental health system. Such a hiring policy, pursued affirmatively, has both its glories and problems. Several of our former members are now full-time staff who work with current members in the professional roles of Thresholds Bridge staff, residential staff, day program staff, and in one case, a key supervisor of Thresholds Rehabilitation Industries. In a few cases, the former members were overmatched by the job responsibilities, became overstressed, regressed quickly, and had to be hospitalized. For a few, these staff jobs were not the right jobs; but for others, they were. Thresholds is becoming more willing to give special consideration to hiring these former members and more adept at actually doing it, and that is as it should be. If we can not accommodate to them, how can we expect other employers to do so? Now we are moving toward hiring former members as part-time professional staff, case aides, and friendly visitors, thereby increasing our number of prosumers. We have also hired members as support staff in the agency, as part-time and full-time messengers, receptionists, researchers, trainers, and janitors.

Other people among our staff have never been members of Thresholds but have been consumers in the mental health system somewhere else. Some have had previous psychiatric hospitalizations; others have not. These staff members, however, do not openly identify themselves as former consumers, seeming to fear that prejudice among other Thresholds staff will detract from their acceptance as equals.

Additionally, Thresholds has organized a prosumer support group, convened monthly by a staff member who has been open about his psychiatric hospitalizations although he never received services from Thresholds. The group meets in the apartment of the convener, and one of its tasks is to decide if the convener should confidentially bring any issues that have arisen to the attention of the executive director. These prosumers are also developing a phone tree so they can reach out to each other instead of just to the convener.

Unfortunately, most staff with a psychiatric history hide it during interviews for positions in the field. Their degree of sensitivity and secrecy is illustrated by prosumer group members who report how they drove around the block many times before they got the courage to come into their first prosumer meeting. Surprisingly and sadly, the Thresholds staff climate needs much more work before it will feel like a completely safe place for prosumers to be open and honest about their prior illness.

Making continual support available at times of stress needs to be seen as an accommodation that Thresholds and other agencies must make for prosumer staff. All of us need to pay attention to the possibility that supportive counseling and other services will be needed by people as they transition from being members who receive help to being staff who offer help. Also, agencies need to examine policies that affect prosumers unfairly, such as the prohibition against staff dating members, and resolve staff health insurance questions relating to preexisting health conditions.

Member Empowerment

It is true that members have lost a lot by having this terrible disease. Sometimes, they are unable to participate as much as we would like or think they should. To ensure that members are heard, trusting rehabilitation relationships between members and staff must be encouraged and various mechanisms such as member councils and committees can be established. As Cook and Hoffschmidt state: "Empowerment is implied in the psychosocial rehabilitation emphasis on building on strengths; it is evident in the focus on acquiring new skills; it is present in the provision of new organizational responsibilities for members. Whether supervising their peers' work on prevocational crews or on community job placements, running 'Members' Councils,' engaging in training of mental health professionals, lobbying policy makers, or providing feedback in program evaluation, the members' involvement is stressed by psychosocial rehabilitation programs" (1993, p. 83).

That does not mean members are to control the agency. Members attend the agency to get the benefits of programming, and staff are there to assist in that process. I do not view bipolar disorder or schizophrenia as social illnesses caused by a lack of power or a gap in the democratic process. I do not consider running the agency the job of members. Members should (and at Thresholds they do) have a role in what goes on in programming and have forums available for discussing improvements and bringing them to everyone's attention. I in no way am implying that members should be excluded from participation. However, the main job of members is to recover from a terrible disease. To get better at Thresholds means to make personal improvement within the agency's six goal areas.

I learned all this in my early years of working in psychiatric rehabilitation at Fountain House in New York. When John Beard first came to Fountain House as its director, members ran the program. It had become an anarchy. Beard changed all that. The agency maintained an emphasis on the social aspect, but it also developed vocational components, and more importantly, it became an agency run by staff. Only later did it move to member empowerment. Similarly, what is important at Thresholds is that staff really hear members and act upon what they say with empathy, love, and understanding.

In recent years, the idea of member empowerment has been taken too literally and too far in certain agencies. Members should be empowered in the sense of participating in and controlling their own rehabilitation and in improving their chance of recovery from a devastating illness. Some persons with mental illness have been maltreated or mistreated or have been victims of uninformed treatment. To a certain degree, this is what has made some spokespeople for the mentally ill state that there is no such thing as mental illness, that so-called mental illness is simply a result of environment or of the medical establishment's definition of normalcy. Some advocates feel this very keenly, negating or downplaying medication, rehabilitation, or therapy, while saying that "the system" is at fault. I strongly disagree, although I also make no excuses for uninformed or callous treatment.

Empowerment does not have to mean denial of mental illness. At Thresholds, empowerment connotes members helping us provide them with an embrace filled with love within a plan to stabilize and uplift their lives.

Parents and Relatives

Once we accept the biological basis of mental illness, fault finding and parent causation theories can essentially be eliminated. The "schizophrenogenic mother," an abomination of a concept if ever there was one, can be replaced with scientific thinking, which does much to reduce parental guilt. No parent is perfect. All parents have done some unhelpful, unnurturing, even harmful things to their children. But that by itself will not cause schizophrenia or bipolar disorders.

The baseline concepts of the Thresholds Parents/Relatives Group are to relieve parental guilt (thereby reducing the feeling of stigma), provide support and education about mental illness, enlist parents' help as partners in the psychiatric rehabilitation of their children, and provide a safe place in which parents can express their own emotions. Thresholds has come to respect the suffering of members' parents and to empathize with them. Their disappointment, their grief over lost potential, their nagging sense of responsibility, the role they can play in partnership with the agency all need to be experienced in a truly supportive setting. Many parents have horror stories about personnel from psychiatric hospitals who blamed parents for a child's illness, who gave parents no information about treatment or progress, but who expected parents to pay the bills. In most ways, parents have not been respected by the psychiatric community, and it has been a welcome relief for them to experience a whole new attitude and approach at Thresholds. This experience was enhanced when I led the Parents/Relatives Group for twenty-two years, with a series of coleaders. Having the attention of the executive director helps parents feel that they were not being blamed or just being tolerated but are truly important to agency activities. The group meets weekly for one and half hours, and is open ended, with new parents and relatives joining regularly. Some parents have become extremely active, attending for years; others attend only briefly, and others come on an as-needed basis.

Half of each meeting is taken up with discussion of a topic that is usually but not always educational in nature. Over the years, we have developed the following roster of topics and events to be covered in the initial half of group meetings: biochemical theory of mental illness, members who are coping successfully (parents meet these members), prodromal symptoms (identification of a child's unique prodromes), how parents can handle the stigma of mental illness, the meaning of psychiatric diagnosis, parents who are coping successfully (parents who have graduated from the group come back for a session), issues for siblings (siblings attend with their parents), creation of a parental climate for independence, substance abuse and its effect on mental illness, suicide attempts, the grim issue of what to do if a member does not get well, the rights of parents, public funding programs and entitlements, the Alliance for the Mentally Ill, and holiday stress. The second half of each meeting is devoted to issues that have come up for group members recently. Some of the value of the group is simply that it allows parents to vent the feelings that they are experiencing and to validate them with other parents. Parents and staff support other parents in times of stress and aggravation.

Through this group, we became impressed with the effect of a member's mental illness on the lives of his or her siblings. In some cases, the effect was profound, a shaping experience for the siblings, filled with resentment of or toward parents and/or the member and pervaded by a sense of neglect and sometimes fear of the siblings' own vulnerability to developing mental illness and an overcompensation in their own achievement needs. We began to understand and appreciate the combination of deeply felt psychological issues that are raised by some siblings of the mentally ill. Truly, they too can be wounded by the secondary effects of the illness, and it is encouraging to see the formation of special support groups for siblings.

Our discussion of parents' rights came about when, with all the talk of patients' rights, it struck the group leader that parents had some rights too. One meeting in each series is devoted to developing and discussing the following "Parents Guilt-Free Bill of Rights," developed by the parents themselves. This topic always promotes a lively discussion. Parents have

A right to survive
A right to privacy and to lead our own lives
A right not to go broke or alter our standard of living
A right not to be psychologically abused
A right to be physically safe
A right to be parents to our other children
A right to express our own emotions
A right to respite and vacations
A right to receive help for ourselves
A right to set house rules and to be treated with consideration.

When some of our parents group graduates wanted to move into a stronger advocacy role in the larger community, one parent became a VISTA worker, and we set up an office at Thresholds to enlarge and organize the network of parents and relatives who could put pressure on the political system and influence the mental health system. This has been hugely successful, and when the Alliance for the Mentally Ill was formed in Madison, Wisconsin in 1979, the Thresholds Parents/Relatives Group was there and ready to exert its leadership. That VISTA worker eventually became the first executive director of the National Alliance for the Mentally Ill (NAMI), which itself has gone on to become the premier advocacy group for the mentally ill in the United States.

Agencies should never overlook the value of parents' participation.

Sexuality, AIDS, and Sexual Abuse

Thresholds has always taken a proactive stance toward sexuality, affirming its value and naturalness. We encourage members to express sexuality in an appropriate manner as they desire.

To our members, this means do not force anybody to do anything against his or her will or do anything to a sexual partner he or she does not want done; do not get anyone pregnant or become pregnant without intending to; do everything you can to prevent sexually transmitted diseases. We use Sexual Attitude Reassessment (SAR) training to educate staff and members in the area of human sexuality.

Thresholds takes an affirmative stance toward homosexuality among both its members and staff, seeing it as a legitimate and caring expressing of sexual desire and human relationships. Since 1992, Thresholds has had a support group for gay and lesbian members. Currently, the group is primarily male, with the biggest issues being self-esteem and self-acceptance. We also refer members to gay and lesbian support centers and programs.

In recent years, we have had to contend with members who are HIV positive or who have AIDS. We believe that all sexually active members should be tested yearly, not through coercion but through persuasion, particularly any member engaging in high-risk behavior. Members who are HIV positive or have AIDS are integrated into our residences and maintained until their medical care is beyond the scope of what we can provide. So far as we know, in all of our programs, a total of twenty-two members are HIV positive, six have AIDS, and several have died of AIDS-related illnesses in the past two years. Psychiatric rehabilitation agencies will have to learn to provide more services to members with these illnesses.

When we became concerned about levels of childhood sexual abuse among our members, male and female, we administered a two-question survey. First, we asked, "As a child, did anyone in your family ever make overt sexual advances toward you or force you to do anything that was sexually inappropriate?" Second, we asked, "As a child, did anyone outside of your family, such as a neighbor, babysitter, teacher, minister, or other child, ever make overt sexual advances towards you or force you to do anything that was sexually inappropriate?"

Of the 952 persons who responded to the first question, 128 (9.1 percent) said yes. One hundred and fifty-five members (11 percent) answered yes to the second question. (The study design made it impossible for us to know how many, if any, members answered yes to both questions). Because of the sensitivity of the topic, we regard the yes replies as the minimum true number of members affected; the actual number is probably much greater. Our response has been to start treatment groups at several branches, particularly for women with childhood experiences of sexual abuse. By the fall of 1994, we had four such education, support, and therapy groups running. We anticipate starting a group for sexually abused males and, possibly, a group for sexual offenders.

Perhaps the most important point to be made here is that Thresholds acted to administer the agencywide survey and, once staff saw the results, did something about the issue. Childhood sexual abuse is probably a larger problem than we would like to admit, and some research shows it is a very big issue. Any agency that aims toward comprehensiveness must address a problem of this size.

Court Commitment to Outpatient Medication Management

Is there any rationale for a court to commit a person to take medication as a condition of his or her release from a psychiatric hospital? Certainly this is a vexing question, one that weighs the "right" of patients to voluntarily take medication against the community desire for assurance that patients are taking their medication.

At Thresholds, we have seen a small number of patients who do well on medication while in the hospital but who relapse quickly on the outside because they are not medication compliant. They are usually the patients who are in and out of hospitals many times. Some have uncomfortable side effects, some deny mental illness, some are quite paranoid about medication, others feel that medications harm their bodies or are not effective, yet others cannot be bothered, and still others are too mentally disorganized or confused to remember their medication or find that medication interferes with their substance abuse. These are the people who repeatedly use public resources to go to psychiatric hospitals, occupy a great deal of mental health professionals' time, attention, and energy, and sometimes get themselves and others into serious trouble. At Thresholds, we acknowledge that people have the right to refuse medication in most instances. But in certain cases, when the court carefully weighs the pros and cons, we also believe that a court commitment to take medication and to have the court order monitored regularly on an outpatient basis is justified, albeit risky.

Spirituality

Psychiatric rehabilitation has been so concrete for so long that those of us who work in this field tend to miss some less concrete approaches that might have value for our members. Instead of seeing each member only as a set of behaviors to be altered or taught skills or molded into a socially accepted pattern, we could look at him or her differently, asking ourselves, "What is it that is trying to emerge from this person? Is there some basic spiritual crisis or issue that is reflected in his or her behavior?"

I see the potential spirituality in members in its broadest sense. In the sense that I use it, it has little to do with formal religion or God but rather with what is emerging from each human being's central core, who that person is at his or her deepest level. I believe we have a biological piece, but we are more than our biology. I believe we have emotions, but we are more than our emotions. I believe we have mental abilities, but we are more than our mental abilities. The inner energy that binds this all together is the *self*. The sum of who we are is greater than our individual parts (Dincin, 1990).

What we most need today is not some ideal rehabilitation goal to live up to, but a sense of the real adventure of life with which we are each engaged, our path. This is a term that points to one of the great challenges of human existence: the need for us to awaken, each of us in his or her own way, to the greater possibilities that life presents. The nature of our path is to lead us on a journey, and it is our life's deepest urge to move forward in this way. Whenever our lives have this sense of forward momentum, we feel an unmistakable stream of vitality flowing through us, which tells us that we are onto something real. Unfortunately, however, we are often not aligned with this force moving deep within us.

When we focus exclusively on problem solving, we often imagine that if only we could get rid of the difficulties our members are facing, if only they could just "get it right," then they could get on with life. However, since rehabilitation, too, is a path, always a living process never a finished product, new questions and challenges continually call on us to develop greater consciousness. We can then experience difficulties as no longer merely nuisances; instead, they can be seen as an integral part of the path, for they compel us to bring our awareness to the dark, unconscious parts of ourselves and mobilize the inner resources—such as patience, generosity, kindness, and bravery—that give us a larger, deeper sense of who we are.

Instead of warding off the challenging questions that spirituality poses, we need to let them work on us, somewhat as homeopathic medicine works, subtly activating our natural healing response. Though these questions may be irritating at first, as they work on us, they stimulate our creative intelligence, triggering larger healing and transformative powers within us and thus fortifying our system as a whole. This is what will provide us with the strength and courage to keep moving forward on the path, regardless of the difficulties we encounter.

When spirituality is seen as a way to become more fully alive, helping us bring forth the goodness and strength already present within us, we can welcome it as a way to wake us up in those areas where we are asleep and where we avoid contact with life. It commits us to movement and change, providing forward direction by showing us exactly where we most need to grow. For spirituality to flourish, we need to see it in a new way—as a series of opportunities for developing greater awareness, discovering deeper truth, and becoming more fully human.

Differentiating between a "spiritual crisis," which seems to have some of the attributes of schizophrenia, and what is only and truly a mental illness is a task in which few of us are experienced. Where one stops and the other begins is a land where few have knowledgeably traveled. We can say that in spiritual crises, people are able to maintain some contact with reality and usually are able to maintain relationships. A spiritual crisis is also usually temporary.

Some people who have taken drugs such as hallucinogenic mushrooms, LSD, Ecstasy, and peyote, among others, have experienced profound paranormal, mystical, even myth-making experiences or perceptual alterations of heightened feelings, energy, love, or light that have been profoundly valuable spiritual experiences and that on an internal level can even resemble mental illness. Fortunately the psychotic effect is transitory, but the spiritual effect can be permanent and sometimes deep and important.

In psychiatric rehabilitation, we are rarely working with people who are only in spiritual crisis or are responding only as a result of mind-altering drugs. Yet we should at least be aware of some overlap and pay attention to both as possible explanations for behavior, perception, and emotions that resemble mental illness. In our actual practices however, we almost always have the genuine article, a person with the biological substrate of mental illness.

What can we do to express a spiritual component as part of psychiatric rehabilitation? Some might find a direct religious approach valuable. The twelve-step approach is a similar way to go. I feel that nontraditional nonreligious ways have the greatest potential for deepening the spiritual component. For instance, the altered state engendered by Holotropic Breathwork can reach a deeply spiritual place. Our use of meditation should be more frequent. Also yoga, t'ai chi, and hypnosis are all ideas that should be tried and reported on in psychiatric rehabilitation. My own favorite approach is psychosynthesis, which uses guided imagery and other cognitive and emotional techniques to develop a profound spiritual component. When using guided imagery, you follow your own imaginative path, following a leader's guidance, to a place of personal inner truth and wisdom. Sometimes in this nonintellectual but heartfelt place, a healing can occur beyond the usual realm of emotions, in a deeper connection to our humanism. I know from my own interaction with members that this approach will not be effective with many. But I urge those of you who guide rehabilitation programs, to look deeper to see if this quest for spirituality is a possibility for you and your members, and then learn to do something about it. There will be those for whom spirituality will be important, satisfying a deep need.

A Comprehensive Approach

The arguments for a bio-psycho-social-spiritual approach to mental illness are to me compelling. We need to become more versed in the scientific aspects of rehabilitation while we pay attention to the psychological issues. We need to relearn specialized supportive therapy and use it. We must be humble about what we truly know and reduce dogma to a minimum. We should examine the spiritual dimension and consider newer approaches.

Finally, may I remind you that schizophrenia and manic depression are truly awful, eviscerating, horrible illnesses and that we should have profound respect and compassion for those who suffer with them. Our attitude and our actions should be heart led and heartfelt and, above all, gentle.

References

Cook, J. A., and Hoffschmidt, S. J. "Comprehensive Models of Psychosocial Rehabilitation." In R. W. Flexer and P. L. Solomon (eds.), *Psychiatric Rehabilitation in Practice*. Boston: Andover Medical, 1993.

Dincin, J. "Speaking Out." *Psychosocial Rehabilitation Journal*, 1990, *14* (2), 83–85.

Dincin, J. "Taking Issue." *Hospital and Community Psychiatry*, 1993, *44* (4), 309.

JERRY DINCIN is executive director of Thresholds.

INDEX

ORDERING INFORMATION

NEW DIRECTIONS FOR MENTAL HEALTH SERVICES is a series of paperback books that presents timely and readable volumes on subjects of concern to clinicians, administrators, and others involved in the care of the mentally disabled. Each volume is devoted to one topic and includes a broad range of authoritative articles written by noted specialists in the field. Books in the series are published quarterly in Spring, Summer, Fall, and Winter and are available for purchase by subscription as well as individually.

SUBSCRIPTIONS for 1995 cost $56.00 for individuals (a savings of 26 percent over single-copy prices) and $78.00 for institutions, agencies, and libraries. Please do not send institutional checks for personal subscriptions. Standing orders are accepted. (For subscriptions outside of North America, add $7.00 for shipping via surface mail or $25.00 for air mail. Orders *must be prepaid* in U.S. dollars by check drawn on a U.S. bank or charged to VISA, MasterCard, or American Express.)

SINGLE COPIES cost $19.00 plus shipping (see below) when payment accompanies order. California, New Jersey, New York, and Washington, D.C., residents please include appropriate sales tax. Canadian residents add GST and any local taxes. Billed orders will be charged shipping and handling. No billed shipments to post office boxes. (Orders from outside the United States or Canada *must be prepaid* by check drawn on a U.S. bank or charged to VISA, MasterCard, or American Express.)

SHIPPING (SINGLE COPIES ONLY): one issue, add $3.50; two issues, add $4.50; three issues, add $5.50; four to five issues, add $6.50; six to seven issues, add $7.50; eight or more issues, add $8.50.

DISCOUNTS FOR QUANTITY ORDERS are available. Please write to the address below for information.

ALL ORDERS must include either the name of an individual or an official purchase order number. Please submit your order as follows:
  Subscriptions: specify series and year subscription is to begin
  Single copies: include individual title code (such as MHS59)

MAIL ALL ORDERS TO:
  Jossey-Bass Publishers
  350 Sansome Street
  San Francisco, California 94104-1342

FOR SUBSCRIPTION SALES OUTSIDE OF THE UNITED STATES, contact any international subscription agency or Jossey-Bass directly.

OTHER TITLES AVAILABLE IN THE
NEW DIRECTIONS FOR MENTAL HEALTH SERVICES SERIES
H. Richard Lamb, Editor-in-Chief